Excerpts from
HEALTH GUIDE FOR SURVIVAL

"You are a prime candidate for a major heart attack! Your food is digesting too slowly. Your cloresterol is building up in the arteries and veins."   chapter 1

* * *

"I could not think of a place to start. Finally, God put into my mind . . . if you knew what **perfect** was then you could test this child and find out how far from perfect he is . . . then you can make a diet to pull his body chemistry back to perfect."   chapter 7

* * *

Over 10,000 patients were given up to die by their doctors, and yet Dr. Reams states: "Only 5 people out of those 10,000 terminally ill failed to respond to diet."   chapter 10

* * *

Doctors treat symptoms. When you go into their office, they ask how you feel. They then prescribe drugs or surgery. When you see Dr. Reams, the only thing he asks is your name. He then looks at your urine/saliva test results and tells you what the tests indicate is wrong with you.   chapter 11

* * *

Heart attacks can be forseen from minutes to months, to years in advance—and prevented!   chapter 17

* * *

People with hypertension are over-fed. Yet they are undernourished, starving. Hypertension can be cured without drugs.   chapter 19

* * *

Gall bladder problems in the early stages are very easy to solve. Kidney stones are the easiest thing in the world to dissolve.   chapter 20

* * *

Through proper diet, the cause of arthritis and rheumatism can be treated and the individual will respond.   chapter 22

* * *

"We have had many who have come here who, after proper diet, have been able to go off both injectible and oral insulin."   chapter 23

* * *

The reason medical doctors have not found a cure for cancer is because they are looking in the wrong place. "I have found the answer to cancer. Cancer is . . . . ."   chapter 24

* * *

Many people have a tongue for their boss. It tells them what they can eat and what they cannot eat. That is why they are sick and overweight. These people are the sickest people in the world.   chapter 27

* * *

Breast cancer and breast surgery can be avoided. There is one mineral that is of the greatest benefit in the prevention of breast cancer!
                                                                      chapter 31

* * *

Note

This book was written to introduce doctors and those engaged in the healing arts of new data that may prove beneficial in the treatment and prevention of disease.

Neither the author, Salem Kirban, nor Dr. Carey Reams is a medical doctor. Nor are we posing as one. Nor do we claim to be one. Dr. Reams' background is in the field of biochemistry. He is also a biophysicist. His research in the field of nutrition goes back to 1931. He is not engaged in the diagnosis or treatment of disease.

Both the author and Dr. Reams are interested in teaching the health message as it is written in the Bible.

Along with his other credits, Dr. Carey Reams is an ordained minister. Salem Kirban, the author, is an investigative reporter, having written over 25 books.

The testing and nutritional information in this book is published solely for educational purposes for the healing arts.

The statement on the back cover: "In one test of 10,000 terminally ill patients only 5 failed to respond!" is a statement made by Dr. Carey Reams and reported by the author. The author did not personally check out the validity of this statement by interviewing the 10,000 individuals. The author would welcome anyone in the healing arts examining the areas discussed by Dr. Reams without bias and with scientific precision.

The author is reporting as he saw and experienced the Reams method for better health. You may draw your own conclusions.

Salem Kirban

Health
Guide
for
Survival
by
Salem
Kirban

HARVEST HOUSE PUBLISHERS
17895 Sky Park Circle
Irvine, California 92714

Published by SALEM KIRBAN, Inc., Kent Road, Huntingdon Valley, Penna.
19006. Copyright © 1976 by Salem Kirban. Printed in the United States of
America. All rights reserved, including the right to reproduce this book or
portions thereof in any form.

Library of Congress Catalog Card No. 76-14377
ISBN 0-912582-24-3

DEDICATION

To my wife
MARY

Who was willing
to charter unknown waters
with me to seek out truth
regardless where it would lead . . .
and for standing by me
when the waves got high.

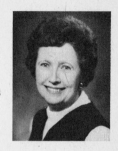

To my associate
BOB CONNER

Who faithfully
through the years of constant struggle
was willing "to be abased"
so that the Gospel and all truth
might go forth in all fullness.

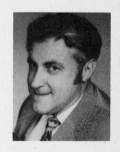

To
Dr. Carey Reams

Who taught me
HOW TO LIVE!

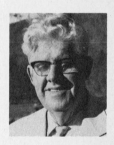

And to the millions who suffer and die needlessly—not realizing that safe, simple and effective means of restoring their health are available.

And to those dedicated men and women in the healing arts, who without prejudice, are willing to use the information in this book for the benefit of their patients—even if the truth happens to be contrary to the prevailing orthodox thinking and practices.

ACKNOWLEDGMENTS

To **Ralph T. Kyle**, who first made me aware of Dr. Carey Reams and his retreat.

To the employees of Interfaith Christian Church who made our stay at the retreat both enjoyable and refreshing.

CONTENTS

Added Observations to SECOND EDITION

In the one month since **HEALTH GUIDE FOR SURVIVAL** was published in June, 1976, we have been flooded with many comments, phone calls and letters. Most have been favorable. Some have been unfavorable.

Since this book is primarily an objective, yet favorable report on the urine/saliva and nutrition methods . . . these added observations will only deal with some of the unfavorable comments received.

A comment from a surgeon in New Jersey after glancing through the book:

"It stinks!"

A comment from a Christian medical doctor:

"Such a book should not be allowed to be published! And I am surprised that a Christian would involve himself in writing this book."

From an anonymous letter sent us unsigned:

"I am flabbergasted to find that you have been deluded by such a clearly Satanic program as Carey Reams' urine/saliva analysis . . . here in Atlanta those who were involved in following his recommendations uniformly came under bondage and have suffered loss of ministry, personal depression and financial bondage. . . . For God's sake and the sake of your ministry, disassociate yourself from this evil and claim back the ground that you have yielded in your involvement."

A Christian medical doctor writes:

"I have one patient from Tampa who went to Dr. Reams and he diagnosed her as having Leukemia. Subsequent to this diagnosis I placed her in Tampa General Hospital and found that she did not in fact have leukemia at all. I feel that in all probability Dr. Reams is a well intended person but I believe he is deluded. Certainly I have never been able to find any substantiation for any of his claims at all. I feel that he is not a physician and is basically practicing medicine without a license and is creating problems for a great number of patients. . . ."

Author's comment:

I have watched Dr. Reams give unselfishly of his time, reading a large number of Equations daily, and yet at the same time, taking time to talk to those who call by phone. I personally know he has made his Retreat available without charge to many each month who honestly cannot pay. One missionary friend of mine spent four week there without charge.

For a man in his seventies, under this constant pressure, I am sure there can occasionally enter into an Equation analysis a human error. **But it must be remembered medical doctors and hospitals also make errors!** Those generally are far more costly as far as the patient is involved because they involve the use of dangerous drugs and irreversible surgery. Coming, however, under the realm of "orthodox" medicine . . . such errors are quietly overlooked. Dr. Halsted R. Holman, Professor of Medicine at Stanford University School of Medicine states that in the field of medicine:

"Indecisive diagnostic testing abounds."

Medical laboratories, licensed by the U.S. Government, are notorious for their slipshod analysis of specimens.

Dr. Reams has been arrested several times on the charge of ". . . practicing medicine without a license." Below are some of the arrests:

May, 1970	Huntsville, Alabama	Fined $50
April, 1972	Tavares, Florida	Fined $1000
February, 1976	Fannin County, Georgia	Pending
June, 1976	Roanoke, Virginia	Pending

Whether one believes that Dr. Reams can correlate specific illnesses with a urine/saliva equation or not is not of prime importance . . . **his recommendations are!** And what does Dr. Reams recommend? He recommends proper nutrition and vitamin and mineral supplements. Such recommendations have no dire side effects. I know Christian medical doctors who have seen the ravages of drug therapy on patients and who believe, from a Bible standpoint, nutrition and natural therapy should be the first mode of treatment. They, too, are harassed. I do not accept the argument that most people delay getting "proper medical treatment to go to some quack." My experience has shown that most people go the route of medical orthodoxy first and then, broken physically, finally decide to try "unorthodox" means which includes vitamins, minerals and nutrition.

I believe, as do some enlightened judges, that an individual has the right to choose what form of treatment he desires for his body. His choices should not be legislated to a narrow orthodoxy that diligently strives to quash all other alternatives as quackery.

Salem Kirban
July, 1976

WHY I WROTE THIS BOOK

It would be a wonderful advancement if all the healing arts **could work together for one common end** . . . the physical betterment of the people.

In my opinion, it would be the most significant achievement of this modern 20th Century! But I doubt if it will ever occur. Below is a description of those involved in the healing arts.

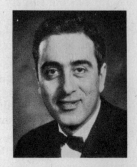

A **PHYSICIAN** (Medical Doctor) is a person who has successfully completed the prescribed course of studies in medicine in a medical school officially recognized by the country in which it is located and who has acquired the requisite qualifications for licensing in the practice of medicine. Generally speaking he is one who practices **allopathic** medicine. **Allopathy** is a system of medicinal practice involving use of drugs which produce effects **different** from those of the disease treated.

An **OSTEOPATHIC PHYSICIAN** uses manipulation for the most part to restore structural and functional balance. However, he also relies upon physical, medicinal and surgical methods. The Osteopath believes that the normal body is a vital mechanical organism whose structural and functional states are of equal importance and that the body is able to rectify itself against toxic conditions when it has favorable environmental circumstances and satisfactory nourishment.

A **CHIROPRACTOR** is one who believes in a system of manipulative treatment which teaches that all diseases are caused by impingement on spinal nerves and can be corrected by spinal adjustments.

HOMEOPATHY is that method of treating disease by drugs, given in minute doses, that would produce in a healthy person symptoms similar to those of the disease. (This is the opposite of Allopathy).

A **NATUROPATH** is one who employs a therapeutic system which does not use drugs or therapy, but employs natural forces such as light, heat, air, water and massage.

A **NUTRITIONIST** (in my own personal evaluation) is one who would seek to determine (a) what is the normal body chemistry for a healthy body, (b) what is the present body chemistry of the individual in question and (c) what nutritional program can be tailor-made to bring one's body chemistry back to normal.

This book, **HEALTH GUIDE FOR SURVIVAL**, deals primarily with the **nutritional** approach to correcting present diseases one may have, preventing diseases of which symptoms in that individual have not yet become apparent and maintaining good health by following proper nutrition guidelines.

Now, I agree, that the **nutrition approach** will seem oversimplified to many. But I know it works that is, it contributes significantly to better health . . . from personal experience. And multiple thousands of others will testify to its validity.

However, I am open-minded enough to realize that all branches of the healing arts have something positive to contribute to society. **No one healing art has a corner on the market of good health.**

That's why I am particularly dismayed at belittling, biased approach (in favor of medical doctors) taken on pages 328-331 of Ladies' Home Journal FAMILY MEDICAL GUIDE.

The American Medical Association was founded in 1847 to raise medical standards and improve public health. To be a member of the A.M.A., a doctor must belong to one of the over 50 state and territorial medical associations. Many hospitals will not allow a doctor to practice in their hospital if they are not a member of the A.M.A.

In the April, 1976 edition of **Hospital Practice**, pages 11, 18 and 21, appears an editorial by Dr. Halsted R. Holman. Dr. Holman is Professor of Medicine at the Stanford University School of Medicine. The editorial, in part, states:

1. Some 30% to 50% of present hospitalization is medically unnecessary.

2. Rising physicians' fees have outstripped those of every other occupation.

   It is well established that **non**-physician health personnel can provide some 90% of primary health care with an effectiveness and patient satisfaction equal to that of the physician, often at less expense.

3. Drugs are widely overused, witness to the fact that three of the four most commonly prescribed drugs treat no specific illness.

Drug toxicities account for approximately 5% of hospitalizations. It can be argued that high-quality medicine can be practiced without the use of any of the 20 most commonly prescribed drugs.

4. Surgery is excessive.

5. Indecisive diagnostic testing abounds.

When required to meet the two criteria of leading to a specific therapy and to a benefit from that therapy, most diagnostic procedures fail.

Medical schools and centers are the pacesetters in creating the present state of affairs.

I have never met Dr. Halsted R. Holman . . . but I admire him. It takes real courage to speak out against the failures of the medical profession in such a prestigious journal as **Hospital Practice**. Unfortunately, such a magazine because of its technical content, limits itself to those interested in hospital practice in the field of medicine. Therefore, his revealing "inward look" at the inadequacies of 20th Century medicine have limited readership.

If we are honest with ourselves, we can see inadequacies in every method of healing art.

Unfortunately, it would appear that the American Medical Association has departed from its original founding goal of raising medical standards. It has done this by exercising a powerful lobby in Congress and using lawsuits to prevent others from championing and testing other pathways to better health.

As an investigative reporter I fully realize that there are charlatans who promote themselves as health experts . . . whose sole interest is in making a quick dollar. I also realize that some faith healers attempt to use God to achieve their selfish goals.

Not all osteopaths, not all chiropractors, not all homeopaths, not all naturopaths, not all nutritionists have the best interest of the patient at heart.

On the other hand, neither do all medical doctors, physicians and surgeons! As Dr. Holman has stated, ". . . physicians' fees have outstripped those of every other occupation" and "Surgery is excessive." Yet, it would appear to some that the American Medical Association has set itself up as a despot who would attempt to dictate what is best from a health standpoint for your body . . . to the point to trying to legislate almost every other approach out of existence. Some believe they have a love for the dispensing of drugs that reaches maniac proportions. Others, even their peers, comment that they place more emphasis on treating the symptom than preventing the disease.

My purpose in writing this book was to see if there were an alternative answer to better health than that presently followed by modern medicine. I believe that every avenue of healing and better health should be thoroughly investigated . . . regardless whose toes it might step on.

This book is based on my personal experience. I sincerely believe the Reams method of urine/saliva testing described within and the ensuing individualized diet recommendations are among the most logical approaches to the answer of solving the problems of disease and putting one on the road to better health.

I am sure this book will have many critics, who fearful are skeptical of anyone who says he has made a new discovery. I, however, can only report my own personal observations.

Their first approach may be that of accusing Dr. Reams of "practicing medicine without a license." The giving of a urine/saliva test is a laboratory procedure and does not involve the dispensing of medicine. It can be made into a scientific test. . .not guesswork. The suggesting of a diet of proper foods, in my opinion, is not dispensing medicine or practicing medicine. No two adults should be prohibited from discussing what foods will be beneficial for good health maintenance. No medicine is dispensed.

The next approach by some will be to dig up some case history of someone who went to the church retreat run by Dr. Reams and then later died. This will be their "ace in the hole." "Look," they will say, pointing a finger at Dr. Reams, "here is someone who came to you with cancer . . . you put them on a fast and an individualized diet . . . and they went home and died!"

What they will fail to tell you is that most of the people who come to the retreat in Georgia have **already** tried all forms of medical treatment doctors and hospitals had to offer. They arrive surgically treated with breasts removed. They arrive toxically poisoned by chemotherapy, or radiotherapy. They arrive missing a kidney, or having had a surgical removal of some important part of their body. They arrive, having been told by the medical profession that there is nothing else medicine can do. Some have been told . . . "get your house in order and prepare your will."

No wonder some of them die! Dr. Reams does not see them first. They come to him last. Parts of their body can no longer function nutritionally because of either surgery, the continued use of drugs, or because of the deterioration of some organs beyond the point of no return.

But compare the percentage of recovery to good health claimed by the Reams method and the methods used by many physicians.

When someone has been told by his doctor that he is terminally ill and has less than 6 weeks or 6 months to live . . . and then goes to Dr. Reams, follows the path of proper nutrition and lives beyond the time period allotted by his doctor . . . with no evidence of disease . . .

Then the doctor, of course, can easily discount it all, saying:

> *You have had a regression*
> or
> *Our diagnosis was in error in the first place*

I make no claims that the methods used by Dr. Carey Reams are the only solution, or indeed the solution for your problem. However, to me, they appear to be a sensible alternative for better health. I believe there is a place in the healing arts for modern medicine, for judicious surgery and the limited use of drugs. But I also believe there is a place in the healing arts for homeopathy, for osteopathy, for the chiropractic, for naturopathy, and for the scientific nutritionist.

And I believe it is time to stop protecting the "exclusivity" of healing for one particular profession in the healing arts.

I am reminded of the illustration given in the Gospel of Mark in the New Testament of the Bible which revealed:

A woman who had had a hemorrhage for twelve years,
  and had endured much at the hands of many physicians,
  and had spent all that she had,
  and was not helped at all,
  but rather had grown worse,

After hearing about Jesus,
  came up in the crowd behind Him,
  and touched His cloak.

For she thought,
  "If I just touch His garments, I shall get well."

And immediately the flow of her blood was dried up;
and she felt in her body that she was healed of her affliction . . .

And He [Jesus] said to her,
  "Daughter, your faith has made you well!

(Mark 5:25-29, 34)

Could this be considered ". . . practicing medicine without a license?"

> **A physician**
>> **who knows not**
>>> **THE GREAT PHYSICIAN . . .**
> **is missing**
>> **95% of his medicine!**

Perhaps this story illustrates the fact that we do not have all the answers. In Jeremiah 46:11 a directive is given:

> Go up to Gilead and obtain balm,
> O virgin daughter of Egypt!
> In vain have you used multiplied remedies . . . .

If God created in us a body fashioned to live on the creation which He had made, then it would stand to reason that he fashioned parts in that body that, working harmoniously with nature, would function properly free of disease during our normal lifetime. Sin, however, has entered the world and thus on this side of Heaven, all are not cured.

It stands to reason that the more natural approach to maintaining good health would be to properly fuel the body with intelligently selected foods. And that the first approach, when that body becomes diseased, is to find out if a nutrient or nutrients are missing, causing that organ to malfunction, and if a cure can be affected in this way by replenishing one's body with that needed individualized diet. That is what nutritional therapy is all about.

And that's why I journeyed up to Dr. Carey Reams' retreat to investigate an alternative to Health Survival. From my investigation it appears that Dr. Reams' just may have come upon another secret of health preservation! And that's why I wrote this book!

Huntingdon Valley, Pennsylvania   Salem Kirban
U.S.A., June, 1976

ADDENDA

On November 11, 1976, an indictment on Dr. Carey Reams was handed down by a Fannin County Grand Jury after investigation by the Fannin County Sheriff's Department and a state health investigator. Dr. Reams paid the bond of $10,000. While Dr. Reams was at the Georgia Fannin County Jail he was also served with a summons from the Arkansas Attorney General's office. The retreat, Interfaith Christian Church, was closed in Georgia. However, the retreat in Roanoke, Virginia continues to function. The alleged charges against Dr. Carey Reams are "practicing medicine without a license."

Or-tho-dox

The word "orthodox" means, in effect, "correct opinion." When Galileo upheld Copernicus's theory that the earth moved around the sun (rather than vice versa), he was teaching against what was orthodox or "correct opinion." As a result, he was sentenced to prison!

Everyone was trying to invent a light source from electric current by reducing the resistance of conductors. Thomas Edison departed from the orthodox and was ostracized. He, instead, increased the resistance. Where others studied the effect of a current flowing through a filament in air, Edison tried it in a vacuum!

In the 1850's, Ignaz Philipp Semmelweiss, a Hungarian doctor, discovered that childbed fever, which then killed about 12 mothers out of every 100, was contagious . . . and that doctors themselves were spreading the disease by not cleaning their hands. He was ridiculed for this idea because it was "unorthodox medicine." He maintained his stand and even published his thesis in 1860.

Opponents of his ideas attacked him fiercely. This long battle eventually brought on mental illness. It was Joseph Lister who performed the first antiseptic operation. And Semmelweiss' technique became orthodox. But Semmelweiss had died a broken man . . . one year earlier!

The same thinking that sent Galileo to prison . . . the same thinking that ostracized Thomas Edison . . . the same thinking that sent Ignaz Semmelweiss to his grave . . . is the same thinking that pervades today by some in the field of "orthodox" medicine.

Is it at all possible that there may be a better way in many cases other than the "orthodox" medical-surgical-chemotherapy approach? Or is God's power limited only to these avenues?

1

YOU ARE IN THE ZONE FOR A MAJOR HEART ATTACK

**A
Prime
Candidate**

You are a prime candidate for a major heart attack!

My associate, Bob Conner, 55, sat stunned in the library of Dr. Carey Reams.

Dr. Reams continued:

You have a tendency towards low blood sugar, a fluctuating blood sugar.

Your food is digesting too slowly. You have headaches.

Your cholesterol is building up in the arteries and veins.

Your proteins are not digesting, and you are in the zone for a major heart attack!

You also have a little emphysema in both lungs.

And you have some carcinoma in the prostate area and in the lower colon and you have a minor hemorrhoidal condition.

Dr. Reams went on to explain:

By carcinoma, I do not mean cancer. Cancer is a dead cell. Carcinoma is a cell not functioning up to normal, something like an old tire on an automobile . . . it will get you there but it may give you trouble.

**Not A
Medical
Doctor**

Before Dr. Reams gave Bob Conner the results of his urine/saliva test he first told Bob:

I am not a medical doctor, neither am I posing as one. I am an ordained minister and a biophysicist teaching the health message as it is written in the Bible to each individual.

Who is this Dr. Carey Reams? How could he by simply looking at a sheet of paper with some numbered equations written on it . . . analyze Bob's health profile through an ingenious urine/saliva test?

Bob was shocked. And so was I. Bob felt reasonably well. His only complaint being sporadic migraine headaches. Dr. Reams, however, in a matter of seconds, was able to list 7 potential health problems.

These were problems, which when they would surface into recognizable symptoms, would normally be treated by medical doctors in a routine orthodox "by the *materia medica* book" fashion.[1] Such treatment would include the use of drugs and perhaps surgery.

**Treating
The
Symptom**

Again it would be a classic example of treating the symptom and not the cause. That is why, in so many cases, the operation or treatment is "successful" but the patient dies!

**Detecting
Heart Attacks
in Advance**

Dr. Reams, through individual laboratory test analysis, states that he is able to detect heart attacks in advance.

In 1975 he warned a man that he was in im-

---

[1]**Materia Medica.**
A branch of medicine concerned with the preparation and prescribing of medications and drugs.

minent danger of a fatal heart attack. Dr. Reams told this man how to ward off this heart attack. The man did not believe him!

Instead, he went to his doctor. The doctor pronounced him in perfect health.

But at 5 o'clock that afternoon, this man's wife called Dr. Reams to tell him that her husband had just died on the way to the hospital!

Why was Dr. Ream's advice ignored?

This individual told Dr. Reams that he was in perfect health. He said:

I am in excellent health. There is nothing wrong with me.

But he died!

Dr. Reams stresses this one fact:

You can feel well and yet be in imminent danger of either a major or fatal heart attack.

A Bishop Who Ignored The Warning

In the spring of 1975, a bishop of a church came to Dr. Reams' retreat for tests. The urine test indicated that he would have a fatal heart attack in 6 months.

He said in disbelief at this report:

I'm in perfect health!

He ignored the warning and the preventive procedures.

In just six days short of six months . . . he was dead . . . of a heart attack!

2

MY QUEST FOR TRUTH

**Seeking
The
Facts**

In all of my writings, and I have written 26 books in the last 8 years, I have tried to the best of my ability to seek out truth . . . regardless of where the chips may fall.

Seeking out truth and reporting without bias has sometimes meant the loss of friendships, and the loss of more revenue that would be derived from increased book sales.

But because I believe in God, because I have personally accepted Jesus Christ as my personal Saviour and Lord . . . and because I believe the Bible is the literal Word of God, I am honor-bound to follow certain Scriptural principles in my in-depth investigative reporting and writing.

Vietnam

In 1968, I paid my own expenses and flew to Vietnam. In order that I might cover any area of the country, I went over as a War Correspondent. I had heard of the "credibility gap." My son was fighting in Vietnam. I wanted to find out first hand what this war was all about.

I wrote my first book, GOODBYE MR. PRESI-DENT, in 1968 after coming back from Vietnam. In that book, I stated that the Vietnam War, for the United States, was a costly mistake. We were falling into the financial trap that Russia had designed for us. Russia was able to spend $2 Billion a year to keep the U.S. spending about $2½ Billion a month. Russia lost no one in that war. We lost 55,000—but the toll in lives and economic chaos is still not over! Thousands of war veterans are tucked away in secluded Veterans' hospitals and for them the agony of the war continues . . . as does the expense of their upkeep.

My reports on the way the Vietnam war was being conducted was not a popular one at that time. But I had to report the facts as I saw them.

Arab-Israeli Conflict

My parents are of Arab heritage, and were born and raised in Lebanon.

Just after the 6-Day War, at my own expense, I flew to Israel to report on the results of that conflict. I interviewed Yigal Allon, a top level leader in the Israeli government. I interviewed the great and the small.

Then I went to Jordan, interviewed the refugees who had fled from Bethlehem and Jericho.

And I reported conditions as I saw them. I saw inequities on both sides. Yet I was amazed at how my Arab friends had used Arab refugees as pawns to keep their war fires burning. And I reported this.

I also reported how Israel used Napalm which horribly maimed adults and children alike.

My stand on the Arab-Israeli conflict was not popular. Some of my relatives were visibly angry.

But I had to report the facts as I saw them.

The Challenge

As I write this, I am spending a week at the Christian Retreat which is directed by Dr. Carey Reams. My room overlooks a beautiful lake at the foot of a mountain on this 44-acre retreat. This is the area of the Blue Ridge mountains of Georgia.

Right now I am on my first day of the special lemon-prepared fast. What you will read will be my actual experience while here.

I intend to write the facts as they are . . . to ask penetrating questions. I will be interviewing guests who are here taking this fast as well as interviewing those who have been here after being told by their medical doctor they had a few weeks or months to live.

Let the Facts Be Made Public

The final revelations of this book may not make some happy. Some medical doctors may scoff at this and call Dr. Carey Reams a charlatan, a fake, and a dreamer. But I want to find out the facts . . . the facts will speak for themselves. I am not tied to any drug lobby or medical lobby or health food lobby. It is my hope and sole desire to present an honest report without color and without exaggeration.

Dr. Reams has many times stated:

We welcome a challenge and have been checked on by skeptics many times.

Whenever one takes enough time and interest to make the tests, we have never been wrong.

Both my associate, Bob Conner and I, are taking these tests. And the following chapters will pursue my quest for the truth.

The Bible says:

Beloved, believe not every spirit, but try the spirits whether they are of God: because many false prophets are gone out into the world.

(1 John 4:1)

The Truth Shall Make You Free

The Bible also says:

. . . ye shall know the truth, and the truth shall make you free.

(John 8:32)

Thomas Carlyle, in an address given at the University of Edinburgh, in 1866, said:

Can there be a more horrible object in existence than an eloquent man not speaking the truth?

To some, whose motives are self-interest and profit, truth is a painful irritant. Samuel Johnson wrote that . . .

A man would rather have a hundred lies told of him than one truth which he does not wish should be told.

However, sometimes even in the United States . . . the greater the truth the greater the libel. Sometimes real discoveries in health are strangled by endless court battles. And the strategy of those who instigate these lawsuits is to hopelessly swamp the defendant in a morass of legal fees and discouragement.

How true is that observation by George Bernard Shaw, when he wrote:

The truth is the one thing noboby will believe.

After Dr. Carey Reams has even given extensive lectures and tests to ministers . . . challenging them to set up test centers to keep their congregations well . . . these ministers walk away in disbelief.

Truth is indeed stranger than fiction!

3

TRAGEDY IN THE PHILIPPINES

**Land Mine
in
Luzon**

Just who is Dr. Carey Reams?

Dr. Reams was born in Orlando, Florida shortly after the turn of the century.

During World War 2, he was a chemical engineer. On January 1, 1945, the Allies had established a beachhead on Luzon in the Philippines.

Reams' unit was directed to head toward Manila to free those men who had been captured by the Japanese some four years before.

It was a difficult assignment.

To keep out of the enemy sight, they had to remain in marshland an entire day ... soaked. To this misery was added a typhoon which started on the second day with oppressing rain. On the fourth day, Reams' commanding officer was shot and killed just six feet from him.

The replacement officer brought his own engineer and Reams was assigned to another company six miles away. Because a bridge was washed out, the truck had to go around

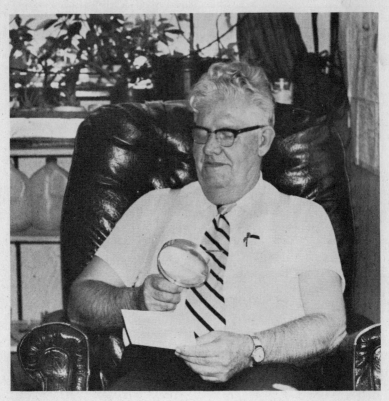

Dr. Carey Reams checking urine/salvia statistics. Dr. Reams lost one eye in World War 2.

and over some fill. Dr. Reams remembered:

It was on this fill that we hit the land mine! The truck was blown to smithereens!

That's all that Carey Reams remembers.

31 Days Unconscious

He regained consciousness thirty-one days later, on an operating table, 2500 miles away from where he had been wounded. He later recalls that he was tossed high in the air and the trees were down under him . . . the truck had been torn asunder.

Upon awakening on that operating table he remembers remarking:

I sure did land easy.

Brain surgery was performed and he floated in and out of consciousness for several weeks and was sent home more dead than alive.

He states that he was one of six soldiers in World War 2 on medical record whose body temperature dropped to the 70's . . . and lived!

When Carey Reams had the opportunity to examine himself . . . he had far from landed "easy."

Paralyzed From The Waist Down

He had been crushed from the waist to the pelvis. He had lost all his teeth. His right eye was gone. His neck was broken. His jawbone was fractured. His back was broken in two places. The lower part of his body was completely paralyzed. His legs were without feeling. He reports that in those parts of his body where he did retain feeling, the pain was incredibly intense.

Any movement caused pain that was almost a deathly agony. He experienced hemorrhage after hemorrhage, lost 60 pounds and despaired of life. But because of his children, he was determined to see it through and not give up.

The doctors said he would never walk again!

A Miracle Occurs

This accident occurred in 1945. Five years later, on December 31st, 1950, in Butler, Pennsylvania, God worked a miracle in the body of Carey Reams.

When asked when he accepted Christ as His personal Saviour. Dr. Reams replied:

I accepted Christ as my Saviour when I was 13 years old. Even my dog and cat knew it.

According to Dr. Reams' report . . . in Butler, Pennsylvania in the Penn Theater at a Kathryn Kuhlman meeting, God spoke to his heart and reached down and touched his body. He said that as Miss Kuhlman was giving the benediction, he got up on his crutches, started to walk down the narrow aisle, paralyzed and manipulating the crutches on a slanty floor.

Miss Kuhlman told him:

Take that right crutch away.

He did and to his surprise his leg bore his weight. Then he dropped the second crutch and literally hurried up to the platform.

Dr. Reams believes that God performed a miracle in his body. He could now walk, unaided!

4

THE CHALLENGE OF DISBELIEF

**The
Strange
Question**

Before World War 2, for 13 years. Dr. Carey Reams was in the agricultural engineering business.

After the War he continued in this business, even conducting it from his Veteran's Administration Hospital bed.

Carey Reams' interest in biochemistry, he believes, started when he was about five years old.

An incident occurred that seemed to lead to the path in which he is now working.

God's providence is wonderful and His ways are past finding out.

In his youth, Carey Reams went to church where the circuit rider only came to preach one Sunday a month.

On this particular day, the circuit preacher went home with Reams' parents. While they were having dinner, Carey . . . just five years old . . . said to preacher Smith.

Brother Smith, I don't believe what you said in your sermon today.

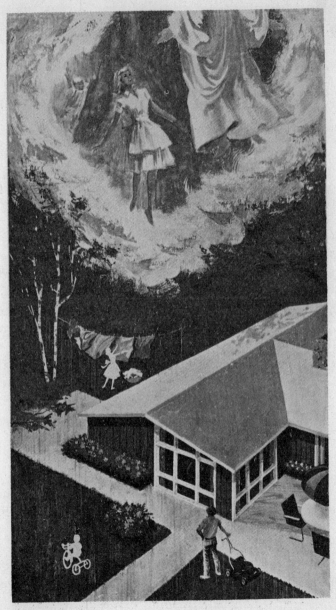

"When Jesus comes . . .
the people would meet Him in the air."

Brother Smith that day had just preached on the resurrection of the dead. He told how when Jesus comes, the graves would be opened and the people would get up and go to meet Him in the air. See 1 Thessalonians 4:13-18.

This is the area that Dr. Reams did not believe as a child.

Smith asked Carey:

What is it that I said that you don't understand?

Carey replied:

Well, don't you know that when something dies, it goes to dust and you cannot put it together again?

Smith asked:

Who put you together to start with?

Carey said:

Nobody, the doctor brought me . . . at least that's what I've been told.

A Wise Reply

Preacher Smith wisely replied:

You're only a child now, but when you're a man you will understand these things.

However, Carey Reams relates:

Strange to say, the older I got, the more I did not understand them. This was especially true when I learned about the martyrs that were burned at the stake and their ashes were scattered to the four winds of the earth . . . and the smoke went up into the air and scattered over the sea and came down through the rain.

And the plankton ate the molecules and then the fish ate the plankton. Man caught the fish, etc.

The more I thought about it the more I became confused about it. Because of this I continued to study chemistry in high school and in college and I become a fiend for math.

In order to get through college Carey Reams earned his way by operating a medical laboratory at a time when ". . . even Medical doctors did not know what they were for." He was one of the first in the southeastern United States to establish a medical laboratory.

Reams was seriously considering becoming a medical doctor at that time. However, finances and medical school quotas made it impossible for him to pursue this career. This detour was to become a blessing—for perhaps Dr. Carey Reams would not have discovered his mathematical key to good health had he been indoctrinated into medicine and treatment solely by drugs in medical school.

Because of this, Carey Reams shifted his emphasis to taking college courses in the study of diet and agriculture ". . . in order to keep people from being sick."

It was during this time that he became very much interested in nutrition.

Failed Chemistry with Straight "A's"

This led to a very interesting experience.

In the final two weeks of Reams' year in chemistry, his teacher made the following observation:

You have performed some of the experiments on the bench but you have also done all the experiments in the book instead of just the ones I have assigned you.

That's impossible to do that for the amount of time you have spent in the laboratory. You have copied them.

Reams replied:

No, I did not copy them. I did them by math. I did expect to be graded on them, but you have not graded them.

The chemistry professor then made the following amazing statement:

I'm failing you!

Reams requested:

Before you fail me, let me prove to you I did not copy these experiments ... that I did them by math.

Reams and the professor went to the blackboard. The professor gave him problem after problem and Reams worked them out by math on the board. (Remember, this was the day before calculators and computers).

Reams, in recollecting, states:

He was an excellent chemist but he was not a mathematician.

Reams knew math as well as chemistry.

Baffled, the chemistry professor said:

I'm failing you anyway, because you did not do what I told you!

That year, Carey Reams began analyzing fruits. And rather than be discouraged by the problem in his chemistry class he forged ahead to a new and rewarding field.

5

THE FREQUENCY OF GRAPES

A Carrot is Not Always A Carrot

With his goals redirected, Reams began to analyze fruits, orange juice, carrots, tomatoes and beans.

He began to find a very great variation in the nutritional value of the foods. He found out that a carrot was not always a carrot because some of them contained up to 300 parts per million of iodine (or 300 milligrams of iodine per gram) while others only contained 2 parts of iodine. This was the day before DDT and additives.

Armed with this information Reams decided to study to become a dietician. In his first year of instruction he became discouraged because all the teachers approached the subject of diet by teaching students to simply count calories. This meant nothing to Reams because anybody could count calories, but you could not evaluate how many calories any individual was going to get out of their foods.

Carey Reams was a man ahead of his time!

He then transferred over to agricultural college. It was there that he learned something about the biophysics of soils. Little was known at that time on this subject.

Finding the Key

Carey Reams however, had the opportunity of meeting with Dr. Northrup of Germany and through one of his instructors was taught the "frequency[1] of grapes."

Everything according to its kind lives upon its own frequency. Grapes have their own special frequency, or molecular pattern.

This is the only frequency Dr. Northrup knew. But it was the key Reams was seeking to answer his question that he had asked when he was five years old:

How could God put us together again if we went to dust and our particles were scattered all over the earth?

This tiny gleam of knowledge was soon to flood the mind of Carey Reams with the brilliant sunshine of greater understanding and knowledge into the mystery of nutrition!

---

[1]**Frequency** (Physics).
The number of periods or regularly occurring events of any given kind in unit time, usually in one second.

6

THE SECRET OF THE ASHES

**A
Discovery
From a Fire**

One day while Carey Reams was in his laboratory, two police officers came in with some ashes from a building that had burned.

They told Reams that they did not know whether the ashes were from a dog or cat or human. They wanted to know what it was because there was an insurance factor involved.

Dr. Reams took the ashes and began to investigate the problem. This was new to him. He had a friend who was an undertaker who had a crematory, only a couple blocks from his office.

Dr. Reams asked him:

Do you have any ashes that you know the sex, age, race and all about it that I can borrow and test and then return to you?

Dr. Hand, the undertaker, cooperated with this experiment.

After studying these ashes, he returned them and realized he had found the frequency on which human beings live.

The human male lives on a log frequency of 24.

The human female lives on a log frequency of 26.

Numbers often get so long and so very great

that in mathematics a logarithm (an exponent decimal) is used. Thus man has a log frequency of 24.

Dr. Reams was also able to determine the race from which these ashes came. He gave his report to the police department stating that these ashes were of two females and one male. The problem was solved as police reported that a mother and her son and daughter had vanished. They were burned in the fire.

From Ashes Came the Answer

Dr. Reams relates:

Finally, I had the answer to my question!
And out of the ashes came the life of my ministry!

In the book of Revelation we read:

And I saw the dead, small and great, stand before God: and the books were opened; and another book was opened, which is the book of life: and the dead were judged out of those things which were written in the books, according to their works.

(Revelation 20:12)

In the Greek, as well as in other languages, the number and a name are at times used synonomously. So, when your number is called—something like your social security number—you will answer as a needle would to the pole in a compass. (Compare Revelation 13:18.)

No one can hide from God.

And some 30 years later from the time five-year-old Carey asked the question "How could God put us together again . . .?" he finally had the answer.

It was in the numbers. And he found the secret in the ashes!

7

RECOVERY FROM EPILEPSY

**Destined
To Die
at 5**

In the late 1930's, Dr. Reams had a neighbor who had a little boy, 3½, whom the doctors said had epileptic fits. This was in Orlando, Florida.

One afternoon when Dr. Reams came home from the laboratory, the father of the little boy met him highly disturbed.

The doctors had told him that their son would not live beyond the age of 5, and that one day he would go into a seizure from which he would never recover.

At this time the boy was having up to eight seizures a day!

Medicine had failed to help this child and the father pleaded with Dr. Reams to help him.

Dr. Reams went to his laboratory and started to work out this problem in mathematics. He was in prayer and meditation for three days and nights. His mother would bring food to him.

Dr. Reams reveals:

I could not think of a place to start. I knew not where to start. I couldn't put my mind on a foundation or anything to start with.

Finally, God put into my mind . . . If you knew what _perfect_ was then you could test this child and find out how far from perfect he is . . . then you can make a diet to pull his body chemistry back to perfect.

And there I had my key . . .

And then by just mathematical calculations and phenomena of the things I had studied about food, chemistry and math, I began to print an equation that a human anatomy should read like. This was four years before I had discovered human frequency.

What is Perfect?

After the next seven days spent in prayer and fasting, Dr. Reams came up with the equation that was the answer!

The equation occupied a sheet of paper which was about one yard long! And Dr. Reams arrived at this without benefit of calculator or computer! Or even an adding machine!

The equation was arrived at through various equation tests showing what the perfect body chemistry should be like. Various parts of the body were incorporated into this:

Hair
Tears
Stool
Fingernails
Toenails
Ear Wax
Urine
Perspiration
Saliva
Blood

And to this day . . . almost 40 years later, Dr. Carey Reams has **NOT CHANGED THIS EQUATION!**

He has, however, eliminated some of the elements for testing because they were repititious.

Unusual Success In Diabetic Seizures

The boy was called in and Dr. Reams tested him. The result was that in just one month the boy was down to one or two seizures. And after three months the boy experienced no seizures at all! In fact, Dr. Reams reports, he was not even an epileptic! The seizures were diabetic seizures.

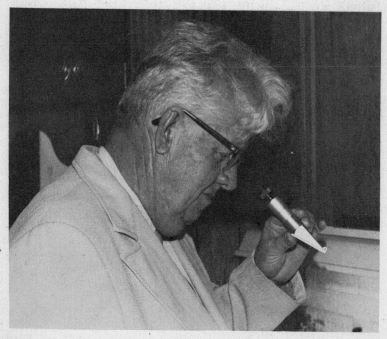

Dr. Carey Reams looking into refractometer. This is an instrument for determining the refractive index of a substance.

The correction of the boy's problem, in this instance, came about by proper diet and bringing his body chemistry back to the perfect equation.

Dr. Reams was able to follow up this case for about one year. Then the father was transferred to Texas and the family moved.

For 35 years Dr. Reams never saw the lad.

Then, one day, Dr. Reams was in Orlando and this young man came up to him and said:

Are you Dr. Reams?

Dr. Reams replied that he was.

The youth replied:

I remember you, but you would never remember me.

And Dr. Reams did not remember him.

I'm the little boy that had epilepsy, and had the seizures and you gave me a diet. And you know I only had one more seizure, very light, when I was 7 years old and our car was involved in a minor accident.

I haven't had one since. I am happily married now and I have two children of my own.

And this was all done by diet!

The little 3½-old boy, given up as hopeless by the medical profession and to an early grave . . . through diet, lived to become married and have children of his own!

For Dr. Reams . . . the answer had been confirmed!

8

YOU CAN'T MAKE A CADILLAC OUT OF VOLKSWAGON

You Cannot Turn Monkey Into Man!

Man has a log frequency of 24; woman of 26. In questioning Dr. Reams, I asked him what the log frequency of monkey is. He replied:

I don't know. I don't remember . . . but monkey is a different number than man.

My questioning continued:

How, Dr. Reams, can monkey turn into a man? That's what evolutionists would have us believe, that we came from primates.

Dr. Reams replied:

It is impossible. You cannot cross the kinds. In the book of Genesis we read:

And God made the beast of the earth after his kind, and cattle after their kind, and every thing that creepeth upon the earth after his kind: and God saw that it was good. (Genesis 1:25)

He told them to be fruitful and multiply. I repeat, you cannot <u>cross</u> the frequencies. It is impossible!

You can <u>divide</u> the frequencies into species. The species are different because there are many ways you can stack the atoms together in order to make the same frequency. We call this <u>micronage</u>. Micronage is the molecular pattern that make the frequency.

Then, under micronage, you have millimicronage which is the path of the electronic orbit that light strikes and gives us color, shades and tints.

Under that, we have milli-millimicronage which is identity which makes everything different one from another.

**It's
All
in
the
Numbers**

Dr. Reams went on to emphasize:

It's absolutely impossible to cross the kinds because of the micronage, millimicronage and milli-millimicronage as well as the frequency.

Therefore, man was created by God.

There is one more important thing to think of here. It is as impossible to cross the kinds as it is for a Volkswagon part to fit a Cadillac.

I came to the Blue Ridge Mountains of Georgia to find out about nutrition, but I received a double bonus in information on the origin of man. Man never was a monkey or a semi-monkey. And monkey can never become a man.

The answer is simple.

It's all in the numbers!

9

THE MATHEMATICS OF DISEASE
FOR THE ROAD TO BETTER HEALTH

Healing
is
Done
By God

Dr. Carey Reams has often said:

I do not claim to have a cure of any kind. We make no claims of any kind. We don't approve of the people who build up false hopes.

We make tests and using the math of body and food chemistry, compute a diet that can bring the body back towards the mathematical formula for perfect health.

Whatever healing takes place is done by God and the life forces in the body.

In order to do a job well in producing vegetables and fruits and meats, Dr. Reams had to know what human nutrition required.

Sometimes hogs are more selective in their diet than humans. A friend of mine raises hogs in Kansas. One day a bread truck broke down near his farm. In order to raise some money from this accident the bread company was willing to sell the bread to the farmer for well under cost. My farmer friend took a loaf of this white bread and unwrapped it and threw it to his hogs.

The hogs came over, sniffed it, and walked away! They apparently knew white bread was no good for them.

What a lesson for us humans! Maybe that's why you never see a pig in a hospital!

Foods the Bible Suggest We Avoid In Leviticus 11 and Deuteronomy 14 are guidelines telling us what foods we should avoid. The swine or hog is referred to in Leviticus 11:7,

And the swine, though he divide the hoof, and be clovenfooted, yet he cheweth not the cud; he is unclean to you.

Our Creator, when he gave us bodies, gave us bodies that balanced out the body chemistry. He created energy out of **anions** and **cations.**

In reading this, some will say,

Yes, but these instructions were just for the people of Israel in Old Testament times. We now have the liberty to eat pork.

But, in reality, your gastric juices, your body chemistry, is no different than those of the Israelites of some 4000 years ago!

While we are living in the dispensation of Grace . . . this has to do with our spiritual life. Our human digestive tract has not changed!

Just because today's hogs are raised on grains and in hog parlors under antiseptic conditions . . . the hog still presents digestive problems.

Dr. Carey Reams did seven years of research before he found the answer . . . yet it was not the research that helped him find the answer to why we were better off obeying the instruc-

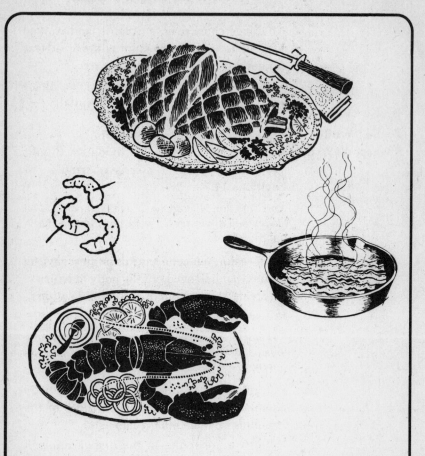

Dr. Carey Reams considers the following foods as unclean meats that should not be eaten: Hogs, Guinea Pigs, Rabbits, Muskrat, Snakes.

The following fish should not be eaten: Catfish, Tuna fish, Lobsters, Oysters, Clams, Shrimp, Crabs and Scallops and shellfish of any kind.

These unclean meats release energy too quickly for the body to make use of them. They digest so fast that you cannot use the proteins, which turn into urea and dump into the bloodstream so fast that the kidneys cannot eliminate them. A urea build-up in the body ensues and excessive urea leads to many health problems.

Dr. Reams contends that the Old Testament food laws are still the wisest method of feeding our bodies for maximum health.

tions of Leviticus 11 and Deuteronomy 14.

Dr. Reams first discovered that the calories in beef, pork, fish or anything else per gram of lean meat are almost the same. There is very little difference here.

Less Than a Year to Live

Dr. Reams came upon this fact quite unexpectedly. He had a client who was told that he had less than a year to live. As an agricultural engineer, Dr. Reams serviced his orange grove and cattle farms.

This client told Dr. Reams:

You've got to help me. Medicine has failed.

Dr. Reams gave him a gram scale and told him:

I don't care what you eat. I want you to mark down exactly what you eat on the gram scale and come in for a saliva and urine test every day at 2 o'clock.

Through his tests, he came up with the unusual information that every day this client ate the unclean meats ... down went the energy level! And every day that he did not eat unclean meats ... the energy level began to climb.

Dr. Reams began eliminating certain foods from his diet ... one by one ... and to Dr. Reams' knowledge this man is still living today!

The Problem of High Energy

What Dr. Reams discovered is that such unclean meats as hogs, shellfish (like shrimp), lobsters, clams, oysters and catfish ... these among others produce very high energy levels. But the problem is that they expend these high energy levels very quickly!

Dr. Reams emphasizes:

You've got to have a time limit on it. In other words, the unclean meats digest in a period of 3 hours. The clean meats require about 18 hours.

What this means is that the energy in pork and other unclean meats is released in 3 hours instead of 18.

Why would it be bad for these meats to digest so quickly . . . in 3 hours?

It is bad because, according to Dr. Reams' thinking:

It's like putting high test gasoline, such as aviation fuel, in a motor that's not built for it!

With the way we live today such quick energy tends to burn out our system . . . causing many physical problems.

We may eat these high energy meats for years and appear seemingly healthy, but this continued abuse of our body one day surfaces into a serious or terminal disease!

Grow Old Quickly By Eating "Minus" Foods

Dr. Reams found that even people who do hard work such as construction workers and farmers, in many cases, come in to see him with serious problems . . . even though they expend a great deal of energy in their work. He states that even some people 30 and 35 years of age look like they are 70 or 75 because of indiscretionary eating habits.

He adds:

We take these people off the unclean meats, teach them what to eat and in 6 months they look younger than their years!

How many people today are eating "minus" foods which may eventually lead them to an early grave?

10

THE TERMINALLY ILL . . . <u>LIVE!</u>

**From
Plants
to
People**

Dr. Reams continued in agricultural engineering over the years. And about 100 people each year would approach him asking:

If you can do this for plants and animals, why can't you do it for me?

Dr. Reams assured them that he could!

It has been revealed that the local, state and national government spend three times as much on animal nutrition research than they do on human nutritional research. In his early years, even Dr. Reams was involved in improving crop yields and animal growth.

By 1968, Dr. Reams was travelling about 150,000 miles a year as an agricultural engineer. He finally got to the place where he didn't want to travel anymore. He and his wife decided to retire.

Dr. Reams never had the remotest dream that he would get into nutritional research for humans.

The key that triggered Dr. Reams into this ministry of restoring the body to its proper chemical balance occurred that year.

**30 Days
to Live!**

A young girl of about 20, dying of Hodgkin's disease, came to see Dr. Reams telling him that doctors had told her she had but 30 days to live. Hodgkin's disease is an advancing, ultimately fatal (according to medical doctors) cancer of the lymph nodes. It frequently attacks the spleen and liver. Medical doctors usually suggest irradiation therapy via high-voltage X-rays to produce a regression of the local tumor masses. Drugs are often used, including an I.V. injection of nitrogen mustard, which causes nausea and vomiting immediately and in 10-14 days, possible leukopenia, thrombopenia and anemia.

She had already been operated on and the doctors said it was impossible for her to live.

Her mother brought her to Dr. Reams.

Dr. Reams made a diet for her. And she is still living! **That was 10 years ago!**

The doctors call her their "miracle girl."

It was a miracle, but Dr. Reams had the answer!

3½ Blocks of Automobiles!

That December this girl, thankful for her recovery with Dr. Reams' diet, sent out a Christmas card. In her card she related the good news to her friends and relatives.

Dr. Reams humorously relates:

The people didn't ask. They didn't call. They just said,

WHERE DOES DR. REAMS LIVE?

I had been practicing in Orlando for many years, and no one paid any attention to me. Suddenly, I was discovered! One morning, I awakened and there were 3½ blocks of automobiles lined up at our door . . . and here we were living in a Ritzy community!

Now, I know why Dr. Reams has his hideaway retreat in the mountains of Georgia. The retreat is found beyond a paved road . . . up a long winding dirt road with confusing forks and NO SIGNS! My associate, Bob Conner and I got lost in the dirt road maze and went a half-hour in the wrong direction!

When Dr. Reams moved to this location they told him no one would ever find him.

But they do! Patients fly in from Africa, Australia, Korea, Japan, Germany, Spain, Italy, England, Alaska, Canada, Ireland, Columbia, Mexico, Uruguay, Chile, Brazil and from all parts of the world for diet consultation and special urine/sputum tests. In 1970-71 alone, Dr. Reams tested and designed nutritional programs for over 24,000 patients.

Given Up to Die   The amazing thing is that, according to Dr. Reams, some 10,000 of these patients were given up to die by their doctors, and yet Dr. Reams states:

Only 5 people out of those 10,000 terminally ill patients failed to respond to diet!

No medical doctor . . . no hospital . . . can match this track record!

11

WHY GUESS WHEN YOU CAN BE SURE

**He Talks
in Numbers**

Dr. Reams thinks and talks in mathematics! And when people started coming to him for nutritional advice, he gave them appointments and had them come back.

He does not advertise. He does not send anyone away. He does not ask them whether or not they have money.

Now that his retreat is well-known the telephones are busy all the time. Dr. Reams cautions that no one should come to the Interfaith Christian Church retreat without an appointment. They are not prepared to handle large numbers of people. Dr. Reams states that 95% of the people can follow their diets at home. Only 5% need to come and take the special fast and be instructed on a special diet.

Dr. Reams has many skeptics. And his reply is always:

Why guess when you can be sure!

**Why
Treat
Symptoms?**

Doctors treat symptoms. When you go into their office, they ask how you feel . . . what are your symptoms. They get a comprehensive case history of your health record. They then prescribe drugs or surgery.

When you see Dr. Reams, the only thing he asks is your name. He then looks at your urine/sputum test results and your eye chart.

Then he tells you what is presently wrong with you . . . and not only that, but what diseases may develop in the future if you continue your present way of living!

The difference. Dr. Reams analytically deals in numbers. He believes that he knows what the perfect body equations should be. And he knows if your numbers "don't add up," you are headed for health problems.

As my friend Bob Conner said, while on his 3-day fast in Georgia:

I would rather be alive and gullible than be dead and a skeptic!

But in my investigative reporting of Dr. Reams and his methods I can report one does not have to be gullible. He has facts and he has a track record!

After the avalanche of people came to his home in Orlando, Florida, it became necessary for Dr. Reams to have a larger area to handle the requests for nutritional consultation.

He opened up a 200-bed clinic in Leesburg, Florida.

At the Leesburg clinic, Dr. Reams conducted urine/saliva tests.

The A.M.A. Moves In

Then the American Medical Association entered litigation against Dr. Reams by a lawsuit accusing him of practicing medicine without a license. Actually, this long drawn out harassment began in 1956.

12

THE AUTHOR TAKES THE TEST

Surprising Revelations

When I arrived at the Interfaith Christian Church retreat center in Georgia the end of March, 1976, I took such a test and went through the period of fast.

Dr. Reams did not ask me my medical history. After my first urine/saliva test, he looked at the numbers that were mathematically correlated on my chart as listed below.

He then told me I had the following problems:

Anyone having numbers as found on this laboratory report would be a borderline diabetic. The pancreas is not making enough insulin.

There is a deficiency in calciums that causes a little bit more inward tension, a very small amount at this time.

The cholesterol is building up in your system, not high, but noticeable.

The proteins are not digesting normally.

Actually you are growing old faster than is normal.

Your enthusiasm often runs away with your strength.

Also, there are some blood cells appearing now in the urine, coming from the prostate area.

There is a minor hemorrhoidal condition.

There is carcinoma from the left lobe of the colon all the way down to the rectum.

There is some carcinoma in the left kidney. It's not minor. It's not major but its a lot more present there than it should be.

Also there is some carcinoma in the prostate area.

And a little emphysema in both lungs.

There is a very little carcinoma in the right kidney . . . not near as much as the left. This would cause most people who sit a long time to have a backache.

Reserve Energy Explained

You also have an energy rating of about 48. That energy rating is based on 0 to 100. It should be up in the 90's. This is too low!

I asked:

You mean I don't have enough energy?

Dr. Reams replied:

You do not have enough reserve energy. This is not the energy you use. This is your reserve. This is like your saving account.

I then questioned:

By carcinoma, do you mean dead cells?

Dr. Reams explained:

Carcinoma Cells Explained

No, carcinoma cells are cells that are worn out but still functioning. A cancer cell is a dead cell. Now, in the medical dictionary, they do not distinguish the difference between carcinoma and cancer. It is all cancer as far as they are concerned. But the medical books which I have do make a clear distinction between carcinoma and cancer.

Dr. Reams then proceeded to give an example:

A baby chick changes every cell in his body every two days. This baby chick does not have cancer . . . only the cell no longer fits his growth. So, every cell in our body should be changed every 6 months. And, if they are not changed, we grow old

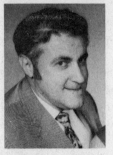

ROBERT CONNER

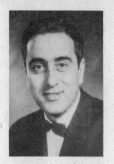

SALEM KIRBAN

Pictured above are the actual charts of the initial urine/saliva tests of Salem Kirban, the author, and Robert W. Conner.

too rapidly.

I then asked:

How do you get rid of these cells you are talking about that are not productive?

Dr. Reams replied:

The reason these cells are not productive is this: you do not have enough minerals in the food to replace the worn out cells.

**Vitamins
A
Crutch**

Then Dr. Reams made an interesting observation:

A lot of people take vitamins. Vitamins are only a crutch. Vitamins are enzymes and the liver manufactures a large number of different kinds of enzymes to keep us healthy throughout our life.

When we are infant babies, we need some of them and whenever we are coming into young manhood and womanhood, others we need. Never do we need all of them at one time!

Enzymes are vitamins and vitamins are enzymes! Vitamins are products of hormones . . . so is an enzyme.

A hormone is a product of an element so it is more important to replace the minerals than it is the vitamins because a vitamin is only a crutch.

Dr. Reams then explained:

However, if you back up the benefit that you are getting from your vitamins with minerals, you can get off of both minerals and vitamins a lot quicker and won't need any of them.

I then asked Dr. Reams:

A few months ago I took a hair analysis test. This is where you clip a small handful of hair from the nape of your neck and send it to a laboratory for analysis. Do you believe in this?

Dr. Reams replied:

As far as I know, I did the first hair analysis that was ever done at all . . . some 46 years ago.

I discontinued it because you would have to shave your head every day to know something about what I needed to know.

The urine/saliva tests give me a minute by minute analysis and is much quicker.

I then asked Dr. Reams:

Now, you have read my report and analyzed my condition. How are you going to correct this health problem?

**The
Fast
Begins**

Dr. Reams explained:

Tomorrow morning, we are going to start you on a special lemon fast. It may last one day. It may last four days or five days. We'll go by the numbers.

And so I went on the fast. While I am typing this story, I am on my second day. The first day was a breeze, but I had trouble sleeping. This second day I have a dull headache, a slightly queezy stomach and I feel a little bit weak.

As we progress through the book, you will find out how I fared on the third day and each day thereafter while I remained at the retreat.

Right now I could go for a fresh bowl of crisp salad and a slice of bread.

But instead, my only sustenance, every half hour is either distilled water or a controlled mixture of fresh lemon juice in water.

But my first real meal will be a joy to behold. I don't care for poached egg. But that poached egg will look like a million dollars to me!

13

UNDERSTANDING THE SOURCE OF YOUR BODY ENERGY

Anions and Cations

Two words are used frequently by Dr. Reams:

ANION (pronounced an'eye un)
An anion is an alkaline substance..
It contains the smallest amount of energy known to man.

Just one anion will contain from 1 to 499 Milhouse units of energy. It is a <u>negative</u> ion. (An <u>ion</u> is a molecule with an electric charge.)

CATION (pronounced cat-eye un)
A cation is an acid substance.

It contains the next smallest amount of energy.

One cation will incorporate from 500 to 999 Milhouse units of energy. It is a <u>positive</u> ion.

Lemons Are Anionic

Lemons are the only natural ANIONIC (alkaline energy) substance that Dr. Reams is aware of. And over one-quarter million foods have been tested. This refers to <u>fresh</u> lemons (not reconstituted or canned lemon juice).

The gastric juice produced by the liver is ANIONIC (alkaline energy) also.

All the foods we eat are acid foods. Some foods contain more acid then others.

So as the liver produces an ANIONIC (alkaline) bile that goes from the liver into the

The Source of Energy

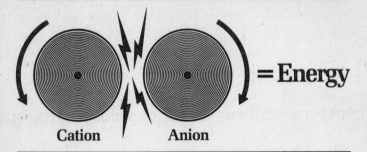

Cation   Anion   = Energy

The **Anion** orbits in a clockwise direction.
The **Cation** orbits in a counter-clockwise direction.
The resistance between these two forces creates **energy.**

Anion
An alkaline substance. It contains the smallest amount of
energy known to man. It is a negative ion. It will contain from
1 to 499 Milhouse units of energy.

Cation
An acid substance. It contains the next smallest amount of
energy. It is a positive ion. It will contain from 500 to 999
Milhouse units of energy.

We do not live off the food we eat. We live off the ENERGY
from the food we eat. When a person gets sick, there are never
enough anionic substances present to supply the energy he
needs from the cationic foods eaten. In effect, we do not
properly digest our food. Why? Because there is an improper
balance between anions and cations necessary to produce
energy.

stomach . . . and then we add the foods to our stomach that are CATIONIC (acid energy) the two opposite anionic products react to give off energy.

Therefore, Dr. Reams says:

We Do Not Live Off The Food We EAT!

*We can conclude that we do not live off the food we eat. We live off the **ENERGY** from the food we eat.*

*The **ANION** orbits in a clockwise direction. The **CATION** orbits in a counter-clockwise direction. This is the vital key to energy. Resistance is created when these two moving forces, rotating in opposite directions, collide. The measure of this resistance, in chemistry, is called "pH."*

When a person gets sick, there are never enough ANIONIC substances present to supply the energy he needs from the CATIONIC foods eaten.

In effect, we do not properly digest our food. Why? Because there is an improper balance between ANIONS and CATIONS necessary to produce energy.

Lemons are ANIONIC and the liver can manufacture those molecules of anionic substances into an extremely large number of different enzymes.

These anionic molecules digest these cationic molecules in our food.

I then asked Dr. Reams:

Now you just analyzed my urine/saliva report. Would a medical doctor be able to come up with that kind of an analysis?

Dr. Reams replied:

Diabetic Tables

I doubt that very seriously because their tables are different. For instance, on the alapathic diabetic table they consider everyone that has 120 miligrams of carbohydrate per gram a diabetic.

But if you have 119 9/10th, you wouldn't be considered a diabetic.

Also, they would analyze the blood and they would only look up certain kinds of sugar. We pick up all kinds of sugar. This throws them into utter confusion because they do not take into consideration that the body chemistry can change one kind of sugar into another kind of sugar and vice versa.

When is one considered a diabetic? Dr. Reams answered:

The medical doctors use the scale of 120. However, some people become diabetics at a scale reading of 80, and on the alapathic scale some people do not become diabetics until the reading of 160! So their scale of analysis is not accurate at all.

This new suggested method of analysis sheds new light on one's overall health and helps one understand the source of one's body energy.

Dr. Reams often states that when God calls our number, we will be made whole again. We will come to Him as the needle points to a pole.

14

MEDICAL DOCTORS ARE SEEING THE LIGHT

Reading The Numbers

I flunked math in high school and had to go to summer school to make up my grade.

Therefore my interest in Dr. Reams took on a new perspective. Math was always a mystery to me ... yet here was a man who always thought in numbers. Number formulas and equations are resolved by him as easy as writing is to me.

I asked him what type of laboratory analysis he made at this retreat.

He replied:

The kinds of laboratory analysis made here on urine and saliva are unique and different from any other kind made anywhere I know.

Each number in the analysis is part of an equation. Direct readings without mathematical computation seldom mean anything. By applying the principles of relative math to the bio-physics of the equation, all troubled areas in the body can be located.

I wondered how many variable equations Dr. Reams had in his analysis. He startled me by saying:

There is about the same number of equations as there would be drops of water in the ocean!

I asked Dr. Reams to look at my laboratory report after taking my first urine/saliva test and tell me how many equations were on the paper for him to so quickly give me my health analysis.

He glanced at the report and said:

There is about 15 to the 15th power. You also received an eye test. And by looking into your eyes our assistant was determining the size of your blood vessels in your eye.

There is about 80 miles of blood vessels in each eye if stretched out from end to end.

The least malfunction of the system that is not washed out by not drinking enough water dilates the blood vessels in the eye and lets us know whether or not nature is cooperating with us.

When the ophthalmologist looks into your eye, he is looking for something entirely different.

In your eyes you have dilated blood vessels which means nature is trying to cooperate with you. But you're not drinking enough water to wash out the carcinoma and cancer cells and nature is trying to put in new ones.

Passing The Good News On

I further questioned Dr. Reams as to whether these mathematical computations could be brought down to a simplified system where anyone could analyze them. I could see that Dr. Reams had a brilliant mathematical mind, but after his death this knowledge could perish.

He assured me:

I am teaching this course now to doctors, both medical and chiropractic, and to nurses and Christian laymen who want to learn something about it for mission work in various parts of the world. These courses are taught in Virginia.

This information has been reduced to a computerized system and all data is being fed into a computer bank. I believe it will take me until 1979 to get on the computer about every problem that could possibly exist, to my knowledge.

I then asked him:

What do medical doctors think about this?

Advises Doctor

He replied:

I find that many, many doctors certainly admire this system and they are wanting to know more about it. They are taking the courses. In fact, I am the advisor now on diet for many, many medical doctors.

We have even had medical doctors come here for treatment. We have given them urine/saliva tests and they have asked for help in their dietary program.

As I interviewed Dr. Reams I wondered how many more medical doctors would drop their professional pride in order to advance better health and a better chance for those in serious medical straits?

It was John Ruskin who said:

Pride is at the bottom of all great mistakes.

My hope is that the challenging data that Dr. Reams has, which have worked out successfully so many times, will not become buried in an avalanche of stalling lawsuits from the medical profession.

For if they themselves would find themselves diagnosed by another physician as "terminal with only 6 weeks to live," many would beat a path up the 2-mile dirt road to the Blue Ridge mountain retreat!

15

ARREST AT 2 AM!

**The
Harassment
Begins**

The night was still. The moon shimmered on the lake at the Interfaith Christian Church retreat.

All was quiet.

Fannin County, Georgia was asleep.

That is everyone, except the sheriff.

Up the one lane dirt road one could hear the sound of automobiles.

At 2 AM in the morning, Dr. Carey Reams was awakened from his bed and issued a warrant for his arrest! "That Was the Night the Lights Went Out in Georgia"—or so the song goes!

I asked Dr. Reams:

Why would anyone pick 2 AM in the morning as opposed to say, 10 AM in the morning when you were awake? Were they afraid you would run away? I know in narcotic raids such arrests come at unearthly hours. But you were not going to run away, were you?

Dr Reams calmly replied:

No, of course not. The 2 AM arrest was just harassment as far as I know. I was not going to run away. I enjoy the court fights.

A Challenge To Disprove

I welcome any study of my method and challenge anyone to scientifically disprove anything that I am doing. Whenever one takes enough time and interest to make the tests, <u>we have never been wrong!</u>

All true scientists welcome minute inspection of their methods. All true scientists have had to fight their way into their existence. From the beginning of time the public has been against any change.

Someone once said that truth takes 50 years to emerge after it is discovered. This certainly seems to apply here.

As an author in investigative reporting, I took the tests of urine/saliva and went on a 3 day fast as outlined by Dr. Reams to see for myself whether Dr. Carey Reams was the world's greatest charlatan or the world's greatest genius!

It would not be a stretch of the truth to say that the American Medical Association, as with any lobbying organization, may be biased because they are promoting a specific group or a method of treatment.

Certainly anyone who goes through four years of college, four years of medical school, then internship, then additional schooling for a speciality in a field of medicine . . . deserves the admiration of all of us. This takes perseverance.

Searching An Answer

I am certain if I had gone through all this preparatory training and then was told of a bio-physicist in his 70's in Georgia who predicts and determines illnesses via a mathematical equation using a urine/saliva testing procedure, my first reaction would be, ". . .

this man probably is a quack."

Many medical doctors upon reading this may, without the sincere benefit of close inspection and testing, make such an "off the cuff" diagnosis of the Reams procedure. This would be most unfortunate.

Doctors Strong, Patients Weak, Costs Up

By NANCY HICKS
Special to The New York Times

WASHINGTON, April 25—A monopoly-like control by physicians of medical services coupled with a frequently "passive" role by patients in purchasing medical care are helping to push health care costs up at record speed, the President's Council on Wage and Price Stability said today.

The council in a report cited the unusual consumer-provider relationship as one of several causes of soaring health costs, which last year reached $118.5 billion, 40 percent of it paid for by Federal, state and local governments.

"The nature and extent of services provided is usually determined by the physician in a transaction in which the patient is often a passive participant," the report said.

"The economic rewards for efficiency and cost-reducing innovation that are characteristic of our economic system seem to be lacking here. Heavy levels of government support have altered the economics of this sector even further.

"Any attempts to mitigate the rapid rise of inflation in health care must take account of these institutional peculiarities."

The cost increase in the health sector last year was the biggest ever. The Consumer Price Index for services other than health cost rose 7.7 percent, while the index for health cost went up 10.3 percent.

This increase, the report noted, now makes health costs 8.3 percent of the gross national product, and the average American family must spend 10 percent of its income on these costs.

On the basis of testimony from Dr. Eugene G. McCarthy, professor of public health at Cornell University Medical College, the committee estimated that 17 percent of 14 million elective, or nonemergency, operations were unneeded.

Dr. McCarthy's estimates were based on a study of union members who sought a second opinion about whether an operation should be performed. Consulting specialists told 17 percent of them to submit to surgery.

Since the subcommittee hearings, Dr. McCarthy has done a follow-up study that showed that at least 11 percent of persons told by their doctors to have an operation may not need it. In an interview last month with The New York Times, He was asked about projected figures of unnecessary operations and said:

"Since there are now more than 20 million operations done in this country each year, the two million figure may be right on the button."

Are the following natural means for good health more sensible than paying high medical costs and experiencing the suffering that comes with most illnesses?

Unfortunate, because many terminally ill patients despite being given chemotherapy, radiation and disastrous surgery . . . die, who otherwise (without any of this medication and treatment) might live!

Dr. Reams was taken to jail at 2 AM in the morning and left there until 11 AM in the morning when he produced a property bail bond. He was accused of disobeying a judge's order. The order:

He was not to have an office nor see anyone to make any recommendations.

The case is now on the way to the Supreme Court in Georgia.

Dr. Reams told me:

Some Medical Practices Not in Correlation with Scriptures

I am not against medical doctors by any means. It is the corruption within their union that I'm against. The Constitution of the United States gives any two people a right to make a contract of agreement among themselves without harassment by the government and without interference by the government. The Medical Practice Act as it is now written is illegal. Also, I am teaching the health message as written in the Bible. I am also an ordained minister.

I then questioned him:

In other words, you feel that some of the techniques and methods of treatment in hospitals and by physicians are not really in correlation with what you feel the Scriptures advise us? Is that what you are saying?

Dr. Reams replied:

Yes, in fact they are opposite . . . I am not against the intelligent and temperate use of methods that have proven themselves. But I am against the methods often used. I, in a rough guess, consider about 90% of medical treatment ineffective and not the right approach.

Dr. Reams states he does not practice medicine, he never has, nor ever will.

Dr. Reams believes there is no legal basis for attempting to stop his operation as a nutritional consultant.

The Tragedy of Cobalt and Chemotherapy

I then asked Dr. Reams what he thought of cobalt and chemotherapy.

His reply:

The cobalt cooks the flesh and it is only a matter of time till the cooked flesh will start decaying, rotting. And when this decaying, rotting liquid goes into the blood stream and strikes the brain, it means death instantly.

Chemotherapy destroys the liver. Now there may be an intelligent way to use it. But it is not being done in this country.

After hearing this I shuddered at the thought of millions of Americans who during one year are taking such therapy.

And my mind turned to the claims that 10,000 terminally ill responded to a simple formulation of a diet recommended by Dr. Reams.

And for this . . . he was arrested at 2 AM one cold March morning!

16

EVERY PERSON HAS A NUMBER

Adelle Davis and Kathryn Kuhlman

Tell me, Dr. Reams, you remember Adelle Davis, the famous author of <u>Let's Get Well</u> and other books. And I am sure you heard of Kathryn Kuhlman, for it was in one of her revival meetings that you suddenly were able to walk again.

Adelle Davis, I believe, died of a bone cancer. Kathryn Kuhlman died from complications resulting from heart surgery.

Do you feel that a urine/saliva test would have been of value to them?

Dr. Reams replied:

I do not know without having tested these people. Neither of these people ever came to me for advice.

Dr. Reams states that every living thing, according to its kind and sex has a frequency number and that he knows of 16,000 kinds of frequency numbers so far.

I queried:

Would you say that, I, Salem Kirban, have a specific equation number that is unique to me, Salem Kirban?

Dr. Reams replied:

Yes, it is unique to you, except the frequency is the same for all mankind and womankind, according to the sex . . . man being 24 and woman 26. But the micronage, the millimicronage and the milli-millimicronage is different.

God can call My Number

I pursued this further:

Therefore I am unique in that I have a specific number. If God wanted to call that particular number, it would end up being me?

Without hesitation, Dr. Reams said:

That is correct!

Dr. Reams can actually draw a picture of a person's health through the urine/saliva test.

Medical doctors have selected a group of people that looked healthy and said they were healthy and they came up with the extremes of what looked healthy in urine and saliva. Then, they drew a line in the center and said here is where the healthy average should be.

Dr. Carey Reams' system does not work on this kind of theory at all. His system works on a theory of energy. In other words, the higher the energy, the more healthy one is. This is reserve energy. The lower their reserve energy the more ill they are, the weaker they become and the less resistance they have.

There are two kinds of energy.

Two Kinds of Energy

There is a reserve energy, which a savings account would represent.

The other energy is how much you actually use—like your checking account.

These two are relative and yet they are different.

I then questioned Dr. Reams:

Now, Dr. Reams, you examined my chart the other day, but you did not tell me what, if anything, I am allergic to. Do I have any allergies?

Allergies Revealed

Dr. Reams' reply was very informative:

Yes, you have allergies. One of the things you have a mild allergy to is white potatoes. Another thing you have a mild allergy to is refined wheat products like spaghetti, macaroni, etc.

Dr. Reams takes urine specimens of those at the retreat twice a day. However, there are some people who he must take urine specimens on the hour both day and night. The saliva or sputum test is taken upon arrival and then only as the picture changes.

Exercising the Colon

Dr. Reams also has an assistant who give colonics, internal irrigation. This allows the water to circulate in and out of the colon at the same time. The purpose of this colonic is to exercise the colon and get it back to where it is flexible and also to clean out the pockets that ordinary laxatives and purgatives do not do. It also cleans out the appendix.

Dr. Reams further amplified:

In the colon there are materials that form like a sticky dough because the liver is not manufacturing enough substances to keep the undigested food from sticking to the colon. The colonic washes these out!

Not everyone who comes to the retreat receives colonics. Dr. Reams determines by

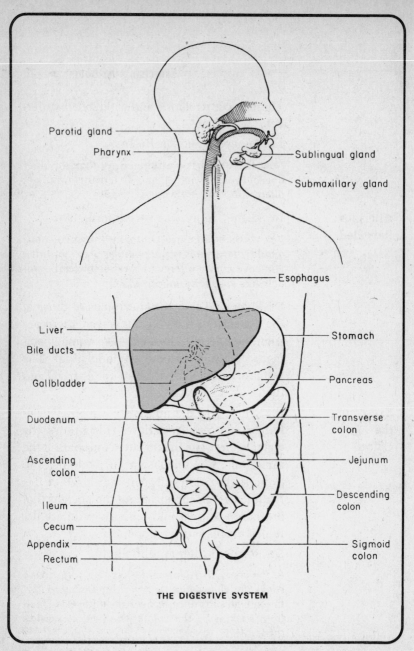

THE DIGESTIVE SYSTEM

Every individual should get acquainted with their colon. And not only their colon but every other organ in their body and then follow good nutritional programs. Most people understand and take better care of their car than they understand and care for their body!

their urine/sputum readings whether a colonic is indicated.

I then questioned:

*Would not the colonic wash a good deal of the
potassium and minerals from the body?*

Dr. Reams replied:

*No, not necessarily. Many times a colonic makes it
available so these minerals can get into the system. If the colon is coated, energy that comes from
foods instigated by the bacteria in the colon cannot get into the blood stream for distribution to all
organs in the body.*

*We also always recommend yogurts or buttermilk
to replace the bacteria in the colon according to
the numbers!*

Quite a revelation! I had a number . . . a specific equation number. I didn't mind as long
as people call me by my name . . . and not by
my number!

17

HEART ATTACKS CAN BE FORSEEN FROM MINUTES, TO MONTHS, TO YEARS IN ADVANCE — AND PREVENTED

The Heart Attack Zone

Heart disease in America ranks as the No. 1 killer.

In Dr. Reams' computation using urine/saliva tests he has come up with what he calls a body chemistry "Heart Attack Zone." As mentioned earlier, my associate, Bob Conner, who took these tests with me, was told he was in the "Heart Attack Zone" and in fact a candidate for a major heart attack. Yet Bob had no symptoms that would indicate this to him.

I asked Dr. Reams:

Do you mean that you have actually discovered a method for detecting heart attacks in advance?

Dr. Reams replied:

Yes, heart attacks can be forseen from minutes, to months, to years in advance—and prevented! Heart attacks do not suddenly jump on anyone. Heart attacks, like other diseases, are caused by bodily dysfunction. The urine test that I give can pick up the heart attack danger zone. In fact, it is very accurate! Anyone found in the danger zone who ignores the warning is virtually committing suicide.

Dr. Reams has in his file several examples (which have been related in this book earlier) of those who took the urine/saliva tests and were told they would have a major heart attack within a short time. Yet they ignored his advice for a special fast and special diet. And, within the predicted time, they did die of a heart attack. Yet both were pronounced in good health by their doctors!

Why Guess When You Can Be Sure!

What to the layman appears to be a very simple urine/saliva test, Dr. Reams makes a qualitative, quantitative analysis. This can be completed in just about 1/2 hour. Quite a difference from the long, exhausting tests given in hospitals complete with a large medical bill! And then, in so many cases, their answer is not definitive.

Dr. Reams' advice is, "Why guess, when you can be sure." And in every test he comes up with answers that he feels are sure . . . in just one-half hour!

What makes the guest at the retreat initially skeptical is the nonchalance with which the entire testing is conducted.

The guest has a bottle which he or she fills half full with urine. In a flat ceramic dish with indentations he deposits several units of saliva. Certain figures are then written on a Report Sheet. The guest finally takes this to Dr. Reams.

Dr. Reams, a likeable, robust man in his 70's, sits in his library in a reclining lounge chair. The windows are filled with pepper plants, lemon trees, tomato plants and other species

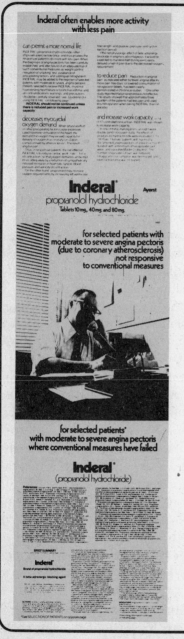

of greenery. He does not wear a white coat (although he has one).

**No
Symptoms
Asked**

There is no long waiting to see him. Within 5 minutes he has seen you, looked at your chart, and told you by his mathematical computations what is wrong with you, what potential problems of health will crop up if you do not go on a correct diet. He does not ask you for your symptoms or your past medical history.

He simply asks you for your name, looks at your chart and comes up with the answers.

The simplicity of it all is difficult for the first-time guest to comprehend or accept. For the first few days at the retreat the average guests are skeptical . . . but as they see the miracle of healing work in their body, these skeptics become thankful admirers. This is particularly true of those who come with terminal cancer, where doctors have given up on them, and they come to Dr. Reams as the court of last resort. Perhaps it might have been better if they had seen him as the court of FIRST resort. Dr. Reams claims that his history of success approaches the 99 percentage scale! If his claims are anywhere near justified, then the science of medicine has something which can be learned from him.

**Pectoris
Heart
Attacks**

Pectoris heart attacks, Dr. Reams explained are caused because the heart is fatigued. He believes this is caused because the proteins do not digest normally and they build up in the system in the form of urea causing the heart to beat too hard each time . . . many times too hard.

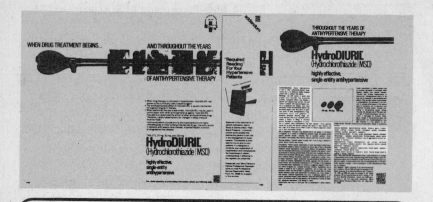

The above drug is sometimes recommended for those with high blood pressure. Note the warnings and adverse reactions. Can there be a better alternative? Dr. Reams believes there is!

Urea is two forms of nitrogen, nitrate nitrogen and ammonical nitrogen. This build-up is what causes the heart to beat harder and harder and harder. This refers to pectoral heart attacks. It is not true of angina. However, the two often hasten the time of a heart attack.

Angina Heart Problems

Angina causes pains in the chest and stomach area. He believes this is caused because the body is retaining too much salt. The salt causes the loss of flexibility of the arteries and veins and even the intestines. Then nature puts cholesterol in there so the blood can get to the capillaries through the arteries and back to the heart through the vein. They keep dilating as the cholesterol builds up because of the salts. Then the arteries and veins, in angina, lose their ability to expand and contract to cooperate in getting the blood from the heart and back to the heart.

Dr. Reams explained:

When this happens and it gets to a certain point, it is very dangerous for the patient because a part of this oil which is cholesterol could turn loose and plug the heart and then the heart goes into a spasm trying to pump this fragment of cholesterol through the heart. If it can't dissolve it, then it's a heart attack. The next thing that happens is that the blood builds up around the heart. And that's an angina heart attack because the blood keeps coming to the heart until many times, the arteries or veins burst at the heart.

Dr. Reams then explained the pectoris heart attack:

The pectoris heart attack is evidenced by pain in

the left arm. These are symptoms of too high a urea.

Dr. Reams reports that he was in Coatesville, Pennsylvania, conducting a seminar in a local church. He was attempting to get churches to take this program and give the health message to churches. They had a meeting of about 25 ministers from various denominations.

Advice Ignored

One minister, a bishop, who was in charge of several churches took the initial urine/saliva test. Dr. Reams told him he was in a fatal heart attack zone. The bishop replied that he was in perfect health and did not believe what he said. He said he felt good.

He asked Dr. Reams:

How long do you estimate that I will live?

After a few minutes calculation, with only one testing and his reserve energy level at where it was, Dr. Reams replied:

Death Follows!

You will live 6 months!

He refused to go through my program of a 3-day fast and special diet.

And he died of a heart attack in just six days short of 6 months!

Dr. Reams tried to interest these ministers in his health message, hoping that they would inform their congregation of this successful nutrition program. He hoped that they would start health centers at their church. Dr. Reams told them:

A sickly saint often cannot be a soulwinning saint!

They politely heard his message and then did

nothing. Dr. Reams' opinion of that meeting is that they "didn't want to rock the boat."

His impression was that they believed the public was not ready for it.

**The Folly
of
Disbelief**

Dr. Reams relates that in one test in Atlanta, Georgia, five people came to take the test. All five were in a fatal heart attack zone. Four of them did exactly what Dr. Reams recommended which was very simple, and they did it at home. They reported back the next day and the tests showed they were out of the fatal heart attack zone. But one of them made all manner of fun of Dr. Reams and told him that he did not believe this, that there was nothing wrong with him. Dr. Reams had tested him between 9 and 10 that morning.

Dr. Reams suggested a simple remedy of corrective diet. He made fun of it, failed to follow the advice, and as a result at 2 o'clock he was taken to the hospital and pronounced dead!

Patients Get $150 Million in Unneeded Drugs, Doctors Told

By DAVID M. CLEARY
Of The Bulletin Staff

If practices in 20 Pennsylvania hospitals are typical of those across the nation, at least $150 million worth of drugs are being given each year to Americans who don't need them.

That $150 million figure was given to reporters yesterday by Dr. Edward H. Kass of the Harvard Medical School after he and three colleagues described a study of antibiotic use and misuse to members of the American College of Physicians in Philadelphia's Civic Center.

Dr. Kass said the figure was based on assumptions that:

— The nation's total expense for antimicrobial drugs (antibiotics, sulfas, etc) is between $1.5 billion and $2 billion a year.

— About half those drugs are administered in hospitals.

— About 20 percent of the disease-fighting drugs given hospital patients aren't needed. That was found to be true in the 20 Pennsylvania hospitals studied during 1974.

Dr. Timothy R. Townsend, a U.S. Public Health Service officer assigned to Harvard Medical School, told how 20 of Pennsylvania's 194 general hospitals were selected at random for the study.

He did not name the hospitals, but said none was operated by federal or state governments, nor staffed by doctors of osteopathy.

On 10 days evenly spaced through 1974, the records of all patients who completed their hospital stays (by death or leaving the hospital against medical advice, as well as by discharge) were examined, with special attention to infection-fighting drugs given.

No attempt was made to determine whether a drug given matched an infection shown on the patients' records, Dr. Townsend said.

But Ms. Karel M. Weigle, a medical
Please Turn to Page 3

18

HEART ATTACK WARNING SIGNS

**Too
Many
Salts**

Dr. Reams explains that the urine test has a "heart attack zone" which he calls the Ionization Scale of blood urea concentration.

A healthy urea level is 6. The zone for a mild heart attack is 20 to 24. The zone for a major heart attack is 24 to 26. The zone for a fatal heart attack is 26 to 30. At a zone of 30, cardiac arrest will take place very soon.

I asked Dr. Reams:

What about eating eggs? Do people get too much cholesterol from eating eggs?

He replied:

No. The only cause of high cholesterol is the body retaining too many salts.

I then questioned Dr. Reams:

What are the warning signs for pectoris heart attacks?

**Heart
Attack
Warning
Signs**

He informed me:

One warning sign for pectoris heart attacks is tension. Another is wrinkles in the forehead caused by tension—although tension can have other causes, such as deficiency in one of the forms of calcium, which isn't necessarily directly related to heart disease.

One of the key warning signs of pectoris heart attack is being tired when you awake in the morning though you have had an ordinary amount of sleep and rest in bed.

Fatigue in the morning is a sign you have too much urea. Therefore, the urea is overstimulating the heart, causing tension and restlessness.

Pains in the chest are not always indicative of a heart attack. If the pain is caused by indigestion, you will also have cold hands and feet and shortness of breath. If the pain is caused by the heart, you become quite nervous.

I then questioned Dr. Reams as to whether he had any information on heart attacks in children.

Children Have Heart Attacks

He replied:

Yes, children have heart attacks the same as adults. About 1600 children die from heart attacks each year, on schoolgrounds, during athletic activity. And there are about 8000 to 10,000 children who die each year from heart attacks, apart from those that occur at school. A child will tell his mother he has a tummy ache. The medical doctor, upon examining the child, in many cases, finds nothing wrong. The next thing you know, the child suffers a heart attack.

Some signs of an impending heart attack among children is if a child is continually too tired to get up in the morning, if they do not want to get out of bed or are slow getting started, and are irritable and have hypertension. These could be signs of other illnesses, too.

Even babies have cardiac arrest!

Crib Deaths Explained

I asked:

Are you stating that because the urea builds up and up and up in an infant, that this is the cause of those mysterious crib deaths?

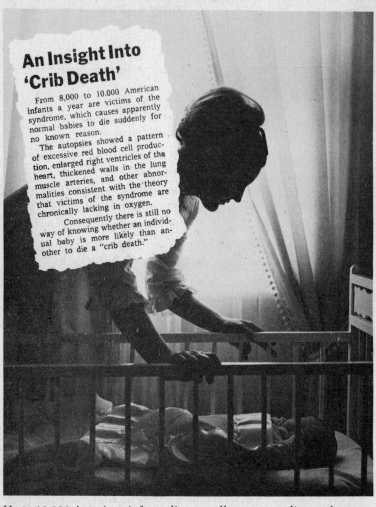

An Insight Into 'Crib Death'

From 8,000 to 10,000 American infants a year are victims of the syndrome, which causes apparently normal babies to die suddenly for no known reason.

The autopsies showed a pattern of excessive red blood cell production, enlarged right ventricles of the heart, thickened walls in the lung muscle arteries, and other abnormalities consistent with the theory that victims of the syndrome are chronically lacking in oxygen.

Consequently there is still no way of knowing whether an individual baby is more likely than another to die a "crib death."

Up to 10,000 American infants die annually, yet according to the news clipping above, the medical profession is still at a loss to discover why! Dr. Reams believes he knows the answer to crib deaths. He would disagree with the last paragraph of the news clipping above. Should not the healing arts seriously consider this? Quite possibly thousands of babies might be saved rather than die needlessly. Crib deaths account for the highest cause of death in infants from 1 month to 1 year of age.

Dr. Reams replied:

Yes, that is true. I worked with doctors in the three largest hospitals in Orlando, Florida for many years. I analyzed the urine of babies that had died. These specimens were taken by the medical doctor.

I discovered some unusual findings. Because of the urea build up all those babies had been in the fatal heart attack zone. High urea is the chief cause of "unknown" crib deaths in babies!

Too often, nursing mothers are eating too much meat. Therefore, there is too much urea—undigested protein—in the mother's milk. When the infant nurses, it gets that urea and its heart is so little and weak that it just can't handle it.

Exercise does not flush out this urea. Actually, if the body levels of urea are high, strenuous exercise could trigger a heart attack!

Not even Vitamin E can be classed as a sure heart attack preventative. Vitamin E is a blood thinner. This can thin out the blood made too thick by urea or other substances. This may delay a heart attack. However, Vitamin E alone can't stop the eventual exhaustion of the heart's strength caused by an ever increasing amount of urea in the blood. And, in fact, it cannot prevent the spasm or heart attack that accompanies such exhaustion.

How to Avoid Heart Attacks

I asked Dr. Reams:

What can be done to ward off a heart attack if the urine/sputum test indicates one is in the heart attack zone?

Dr. Reams replied:

It's rather simple. That's why people find it hard to believe. You have to cleanse your system and *wash out the excess urea. You do this by drinking distilled water. I do not recommend tap water. I do not recommend spring water. I specifically suggest <u>distilled</u> water.*

You should drink about half your weight in ounces per day. A person who weighs 160 pounds, should drink 80 ounces (10 glasses at 8 ounces per glass). One who weighs 120 pounds, should drink 60 ounces of distilled water. Low blood sugar patients should be under supervision in regard to water intake.

I asked:

What is your first approach to an individual's problem?

Dr. Reams outlined:

First we get their body chemistry back to the zone we call the perfect zone. In the urine/saliva test, we measure 5 different variables:

    (1) The acidity of the urine and saliva;
    (2) The amount of sugars and all carbohydrates in the urine;
    (3) The salts in the urine;
    (4) The number of dead cells excreted per 100 lbs. of body weight;
    (5) The amount of urea in the urine.

Our perfect profile is a computation of 6.40.

No Shotgun Approach to Vitamin Consumption

Dr. Reams does not advocate taking a multitude of vitamin pills a day. He does suggest certain types of vitamins to those who have low energy. But once that energy gets back to normal, he finds they don't need them. Actually, he believes, in many cases, the taking of vitamins can aggravate one's condition.

I asked:

Is Vitamin C one of these vitamins?

He stated:

Yes, Vitamin C is one of those vitamins that can aggravate a condition. Vitamin D is another. Vitamin D often slows down digestion. If you have an acid system, you need Vitamin D, but if you have an alkaline system, you do not need Vitamin D. We should have a slightly acid balance. If we have this balance, the taking of Vitamin C would hinder this proper balance. Vitamin D raises your calcium availability and Vitamin C lowers your calcium availability.

Along with the drinking of distilled water, Dr. Reams creates for each patient a custom-prepared diet. This differs with each individual. There is no standard diet that would apply to any group of people.

Dr. Reams encourages:

We need to eat as much fresh vegetables right out of the garden so we don't have to buy the food with all the additives that are put in them.

I would never suggest you eat ice cream. It's embalmed! That is, unless you can buy it natural, without additives.

Two key variables for heart attack are the absolute levels of urea and salts in the urine. Too much of either, urea or salts, is symptomatic of a coming heart attack.

A side benefit of Dr. Reams' guidelines of drinking distilled water at set intervals and following his nutritional diet is that one's personality changes.

Marriages Improve

Tension dissolves. Wives often comment on the personality improvement in their husbands (and vice-versa) once the urea problem has been brought under control. Married couples who have been embroiled in continual arguments and thinking of divorce, suddenly are at peace once again!

Dr. Reams has a history of success in the prevention of heart attacks. Yet countless numbers ignore his simple answer . . . and according to him, they die prematurely!

A WORD OF EXPLANATION

Dr. Carey Reams has a mathematical equation expressing a healthy level of urea.

All of these minor heart attacks, major heart attacks, as well as a zone for cardiac arrest . . . are brought about, according to Dr. Reams, because of the body not assimilating the proteins in our foods. These proteins turn to urea and cause excessive amounts of stress and illness and death. There are exceptions to these rules depending upon the reserve energy.

Dr. Reams believes if the high urea was the only thing that was wrong with the body chemistry, this numbers evaluation for heart disease would be accurate. However, if there are other problems, these numbers must be read in correlation with the entire equation, and may indicate other health problems.

There are two kinds of urea, the soluble and the insoluble. The insoluble urea, Dr. Reams believes, does not over stimulate the heart.

Therefore urea levels mentioned on page 86 of this book should be read with the above explanation in mind.

19

HIGH BLOOD PRESSURE . . . AND HOW TO AVOID IT

**Origins
of High
Blood Pressure**

High blood pressure has two main causes . . . one is pressure from within and the other is pressure from without.

Dr. Reams relates:

Pressure from within develops when a person has a chip on his shoulder, hates somebody and wants revenge for one thing or another.

Pressure from without is caused by scar tissue and swellings in the tissues that press inward on blood vessels. When this occurs, the heart has to pump harder to get the blood to the capillaries. The swelling occurs because old cells are dying and need to be replaced. They do not produce enough energy. The body simply lacks the raw materials to build new cells. The old cells start to decay. Then they swell with carbon dioxide. Therefore, they retain too much water.

In our urine test, we check for the dead and carcinoma cell count in the urine. This tells us how well the body is throwing off the old cells and building new ones.

Dr. Reams' method of testing can detect a tendency towards high blood pressure and his dietary recommendations can correct this. Dr. Reams has been able to bring one's blood pressure back to normal with diet and with chiropractic adjustments.

**Foods
Digest
too Slowly**

Hypertension is not necessarily high blood pressure. Dr. Reams believes there is only one cause of hypertension that he has ever found—and that is when food digests too

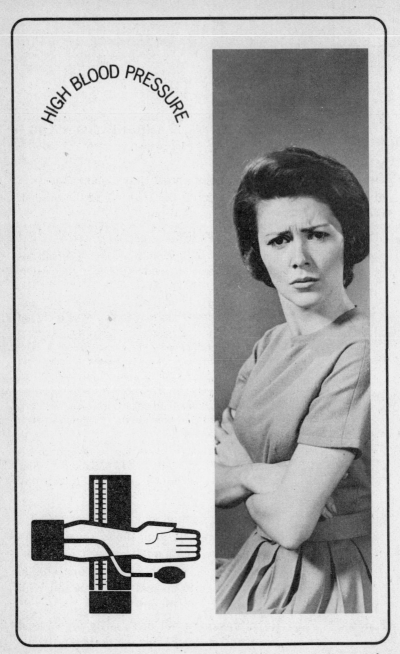

HIGH BLOOD PRESSURE

Are drugs the real answer to controlling hypertension? Or can it be reduced safely through proper nutrition?

slowly and causes constipation.

Dr. Reams explains:

The proteins in these cases do not digest normally. They turn to urea. This overworks the heart. You will find these people worn out and tired all the time.

People with hypertension are over-fed. They are undernourished, starving and miserable.

Hypertension usually causes meanness, irritability and nastiness, although this is not always the case. There are some people with hypertension who do not even know it. And because they have mastered their tension by the grace of God they are under complete self-control. However, even this does not always prevent heart attacks.

Children and Hypertension

I then asked Dr. Reams:

Have you had any experience with children and hypertension?

He quickly replied:

Oh, yes!

One example involved two young brothers, ages 9 and 12. They had been expelled from three schools. The parents were told if they were expelled again, they would be sent to a reformatory.

We ran tests on them. We saw very quickly that they were undernourished and constipated. Actually, they were starving to death. Yet by outward appearances they looked healthy!

While I was conducting these tests, these children were all over my office. They made a mess of it in quick order!

I asked:

What did you do?

Dr Reams replied:

I wrote out a program of menus for the boys and

recommended a series of colonics to get their bowels unclogged. These kids were living on hamburgers. I eliminated this.

I was surprised and asked:

What? You mean to tell me you eliminated the all-American hamburger . . . and I suppose french fries, too? Aren't they as patriotic as your local friendly undertaker? What's there to eat if you take a child off hamburgers?

Dr. Reams smiled:

Yes, I took these children off of hamburgers and french fries. There are many, good, wholesome, nutritional foods a child can eat . . . and like immensely, too, once his tastebuds get acclimated. Then he will prefer these foods above the hamburgers and french fries he ate previously.

Dr. Reams then gave his opinion on meats and peanut butter:

Children under 12 years of age should not have meats of any kind. And children under 8 should not eat nuts or nut butters!

If you give these foods too early in life, a child's digestive juices are not strong enough to handle them. And when you give a child foods he can't digest, it will make him irritable and tense. It will also cause him to have digestive problems.

I then asked:

Well, what happened when you took these two ruffians off of hamburgers and the 'no-no' foods?

Dr. Reams replied:

In three weeks they were no longer wild ruffians but pleasant little gentlemen.

Quite amusingly, the nine-year-old said:

Doctor, I want to ask you a question. Before I went on my diet, my teacher was an old hag. But now she's the sweetest teacher in the world. How did my diet help my teacher?

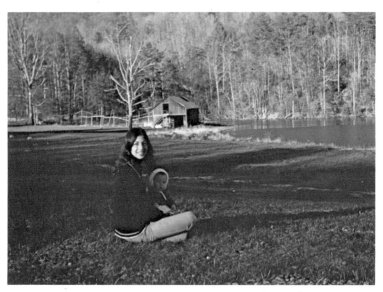

Doreen and little Joshua Frick enjoy sunset at Blue Ridge retreat.

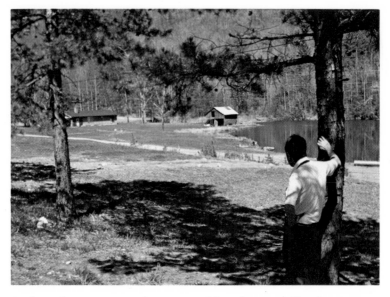
Author relaxes at retreat between writing chapters of book.

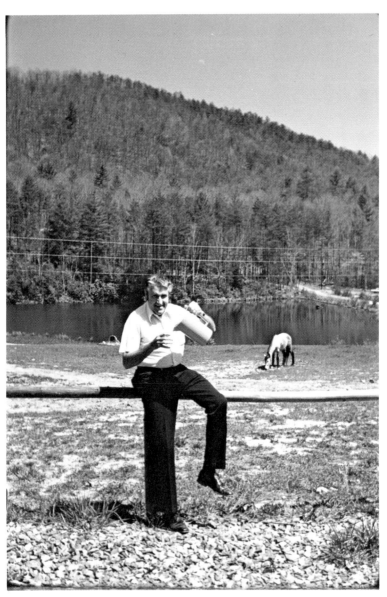

Bob Conner prepares to drink 4 ounces of his lemon water at retreat.

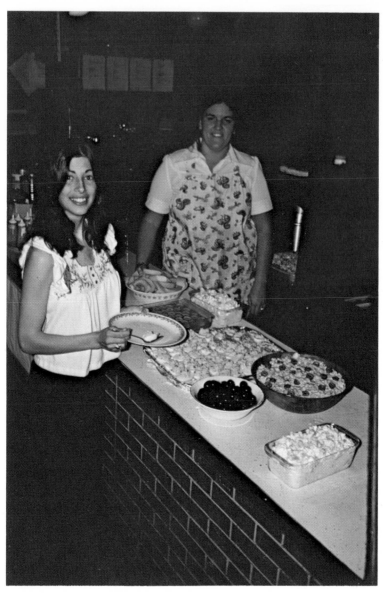

Doreen Frick enjoys Sunday salad specials at retreat.

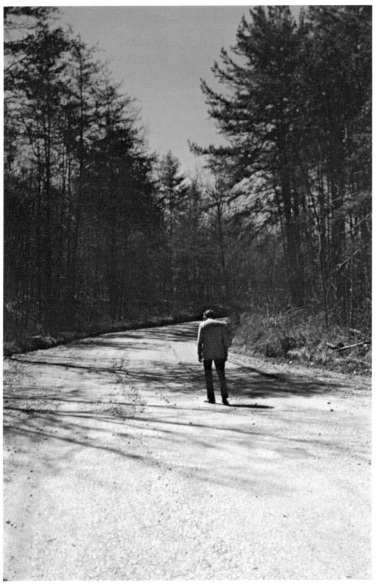

Here is where the paved road ends and the dirt road begins to the Reams retreat. The dirt road has many branches and there are no signs. But the determined finally find the retreat location.

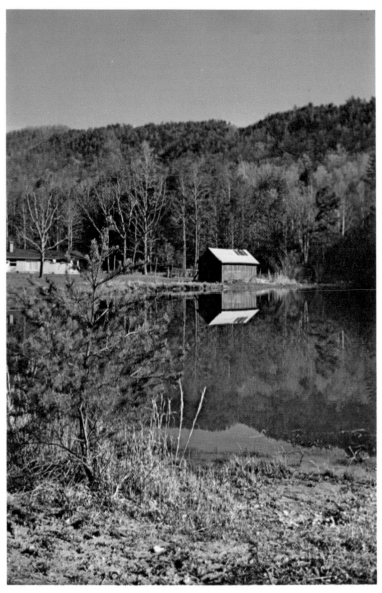

One of the many picturesque signs on the 44-acre retreat.

MEDICAL CARE — A GROWING MYSTERY

MEDICAL MANPOWER IS INCREASING FASTER THAN POPULATION

1966-1976

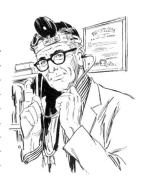

U.S. population	UP 17%
Physicians in practice	UP 22%
Professional nurses in practice	UP 44%
Nonprofessional nurses*	UP 63%
X-ray technologists	UP 56%
Clinical-laboratory workers	UP 70%
Dentists	UP 13%
Dental assistants	UP 32%
Dental hygienists	UP 54%

*Practical nurses, aides, orderlies, attendants

MORE MONEY IS BEING SPENT FOR HEALTH SERVICES

Spending for Hospitalization, Physicians' and Dentists' Services

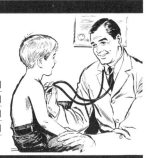

1955	$11 BILLION
1960	$17 BILLION
1965	$25 BILLION
1976	$120 BILLION

MEDICAL SERVICES HAVE EXPANDED

1960-76

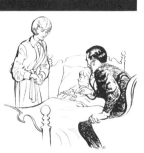

Physician-directed services (all services billed to patients by private physicians, including services of medical assistants and laboratories)	UP 81%
Dentist-directed services	UP 47%
Hospital services	UP 65%

AND YET—Many American families can't find a doctor when they need one, can't get a nurse at any price, can't get an appointment to have eyes or teeth checked without waiting weeks or months. People often run into hurried and slipshod treatment in hospitals and clinics. And the situation is getting worse in many places.

Basic data: National Advisory Commission on Health Manpower
Copyright 1976 Salem Kirban, Inc.

Above is a warrant issued to author in Columbus, Ohio, May 26, 1976. The author was taken out of the lecture Hall at Holiday Inn in the middle of his "Bible and Health" lecture. He was held four hours in the Columbus jail until a bond could be arranged. Three of his associates were subjected to the same treatment. The charges were dismissed in September, 1976.

WEATHER
Partly cloudy tonight, low near 56. High Friday mild 70s.
(Map, Data on Page D-3)

The Columbus Dispatch

CAPITAL
EDITION
Associated Press, United Press International and Copley News Services

72 Pages   *OHIO'S GREATEST HOME NEWSPAPER*   4 Sections

VOL. 105, NO. 332   COLUMBUS, OHIO 43216, THURSDAY, MAY 27, 1976   15 Cents

Lecturer Is Arrested During 'Health' Speech

Salem Kirban was lecturing "on the health laws of the Bible" when a State Medical Board investigator and a Columbus policeman arrested him Wednesday night.

Kirban was presenting his health seminar to about 50 paying customers in the ballroom of the Holiday Inn at 1212 E. Dublin-Granville Rd. about 8:05 p.m. when he was arrested, the investigator said.

KIRBAN AND THREE associates were charged with practicing medicine without a certificate. The associates were arrested in a room at the motel, investigator Jerry C. McDaniel said.

Kirban, 51, of Beth Hyn, Pa., claims he has written 26 books which are sold predominantly in "Christian bookstores" and said he and his associates broke no laws.

McDaniel charged the four broke the law by being involved in the so-called analysis of urine and saliva samples taken (in private) from the customers who paid $3 each to attend the seminar.

MANY OF THE customers were lured to the seminar by a four-page flier that promises nothing but implies that persons who attend the seminar may obtain relief from all sorts of diseases and ailments — from heart trouble and cancer to quick tempers and that "dragged out" feeling.

McDaniel was lured to the seminar by a flier, given to him by someone who received it in the mail, the investigator said.

"I paid my $3 to someone in the lobby and was directed to a second floor room, where they took a urine and saliva sample and told me it would give a partial diagnosis," McDaniel said.

McDaniel and Police Officer Edward K. Kallay Jr. arrested Kirban when he was 35 minutes into his lecture.

"I WAS GRABBED by the arm and pulled out of the ballroom," Kirban protested later. He complained he was not even "allowed to return to the meeting to explain what happened."

Kirban has lectured in all 50 states without previous incident, he said.

He added that the urine and saliva analysis, sponsored by his religious organization, Second Coming Inc., was initiated only two months ago.

The flier, distributed by Second Coming Inc., claims a unique analysis is made of specimens of urine and saliva. "These test numbers (obtained in the analysis) produce a mathematical equation which gives a profile of your very own body chemistry."

THE FLIER STATES the analysis "conducted by Dr. Carey Reams . . . can provide you with more accurate information on your health than can a physical examination."

Reams "is NOT a medical doctor," the flier says. It claims Reams is a biochemist and biophysicist and "a mathematical genius."

Kirban said that when an individual understands the chemistry of his body, he is urged to "follow the health laws of the Bible, especially in regards to fasting."

Above is a newspaper report of the incident that appeared in the Columbus newspaper the following day.

And justice turned back, and righteousness stands far away; For truth stumbled in the street, And uprightness cannot enter.

(Isaiah 59:14)

HIGH COST OF ILLNESS

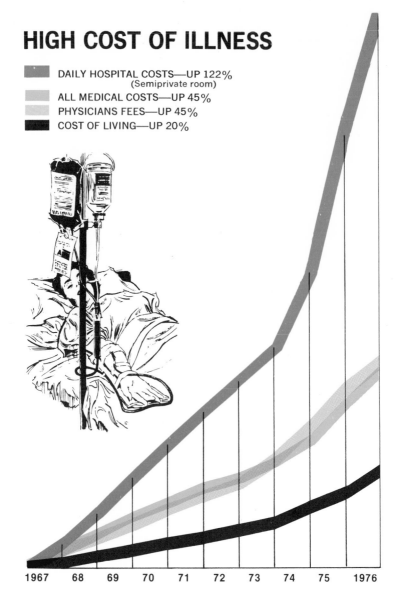

DAILY HOSPITAL COSTS—UP 122%
(Semiprivate room)
ALL MEDICAL COSTS—UP 45%
PHYSICIANS FEES—UP 45%
COST OF LIVING—UP 20%

1967 68 69 70 71 72 73 74 75 1976

Each year 40 million Americans go into a general hospital, where they spend an average of 7 days and get a bill of $1,017.00.

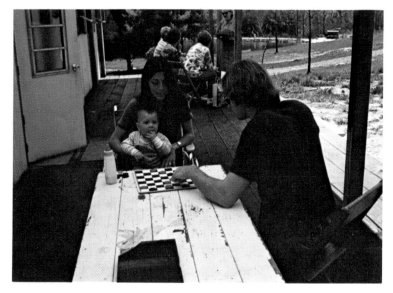

A moment of relaxation. Even babies come to the retreat for an individualized diet recommendation.

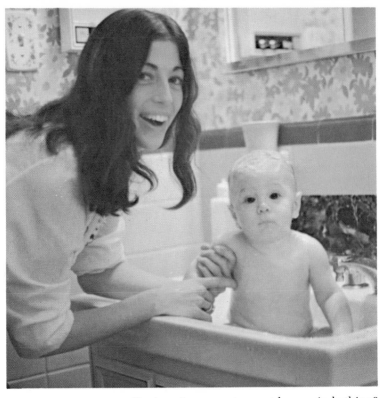

Do Americans use too much soap in bathing?

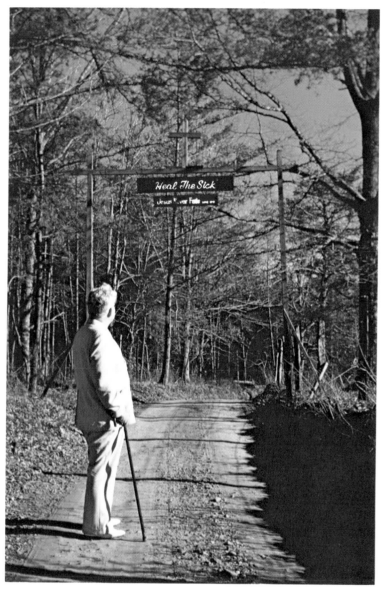

Dr. Carey Reams devotes his entire time in bringing the health message as found in the Bible. This sign is what guests see upon leaving the retreat. Most leave relaxed, refreshed and rejuvenated.

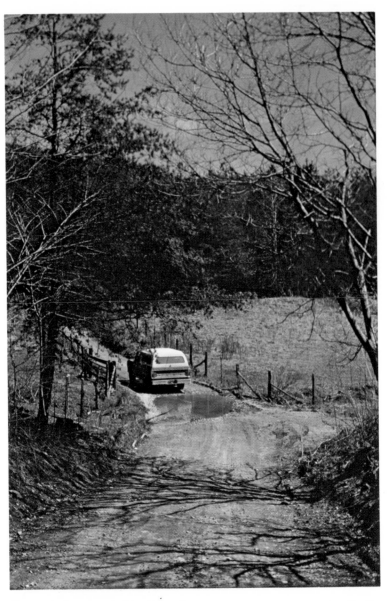

To reach the retreat of Dr. Carey Reams one must go over a 2½ mile dirt road which includes driving through a small stream!

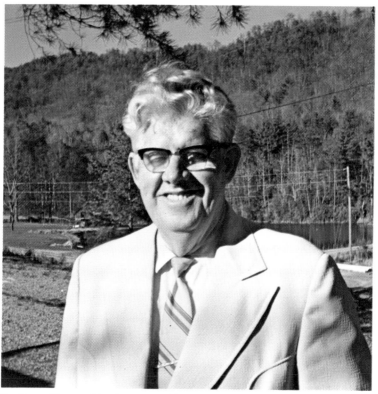
Dr. Carey Reams, biochemist and biophysicist. Minister and founder of the Interfaith Christian Church.

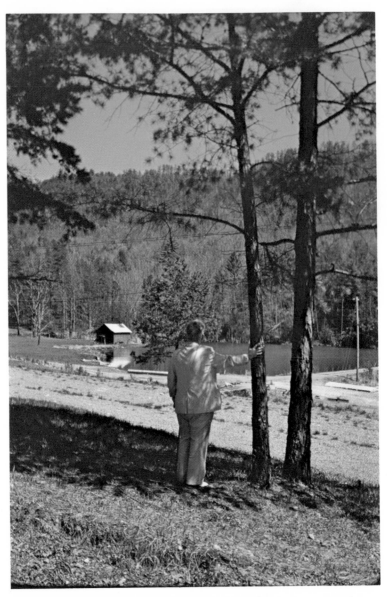

Dr. Carey Reams in a moment of reflection at his 44-acre retreat.

20

THE GALL OF GALLSTONES
AND THE SIMPLICITY OF KIDNEY STONES

Incidence Higher in Women

In most cases gallstones are single or multiple hard nodules of cholesterol, which in some people apparently precipitate into solids in the gall bladder during the process of concentration of bile. Other stones may contain calcium salts. These stones tend to form in middle life and are most commonly found in overweight women who have had one or more pregnancies. Incidence is higher in women than in men.

Some people live out their lives not realizing they have gallstones. Most common symptoms of the presence of gallstones is:

(1) Excessive flatulence;
(2) Belching;
(3) Acid indigestion;
(4) Rather vague complaints of feeling overstuffed and uncomfortable, especially after meals.

When the gallstones become wedged or impacted in the cystic duct, the most frequent symptom is severe pain. This is usually found high in the abdomen, beginning abruptly several hours after a heavy meal.

The pains come in waves. They appear to increase to agonizing proportions, then they ease off, only to recur again. Jaundice may appear temporarily because of the backup of bile.

Who Shall Live,
Who Shall Die?

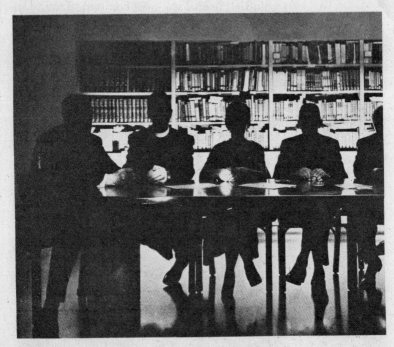

The end of the road for those who lose their kidneys is becoming
dependent on a machine. Anyone who is on dialysis knows the trials of
such dependence. Isn't prevention through intelligent nutrition a better
answer?

The gall bladder is located at just the most inaccessible place one could find in the human body for the surgeon's fingers to reach.

Avoiding Major Surgery

If one can correct the gall bladder condition before it reaches a non-reversible stage, one will be able to avoid major surgery.

In the first urine/saliva test, Dr. Reams cannot detect an enlarged gall bladder. But after three or four consecutive tests it will pick up this malady. The gall bladder stretches so thinly that it does not at first give off enough energy to pick it up. But further testing does reveal the problem.

I asked Dr. Reams:

Many people have their gall bladder removed by surgery. But I have read that many times after this operation, these people have the same symptoms.

Dr. Reams affirmed:

Many times a gall bladder is taken out when it does not need to be removed.

But when a gall bladder gets to the stage where it holds two quarts (more or less) of liver bile and it becomes so heavy that it crimps the tube and it goes into the stomach and it ferments . . . and only when they lay down can it flow into their system . . . and they have to sit up to keep from being in misery, there is nothing else to do but have it surgically removed.

I questioned:

Have you seen people here with gall bladder problems become better with your diet recommendations?

Dr. Reams continued:

Yes! Gall bladder problems in the early stages are very easy to solve, but after they get large enough to hold a pint of fluid, it is very difficult to get them to go back to normal size.

Kidney Stones
Easy
to Dissolve

I asked:

What about kidney stones?

Dr. Reams answered:

Kidney stones are the easiest thing in the world to dissolve. They are no problem at all.

There are two kinds of kidney stones. There is one I would call the pink one, which is an alkaline stone.

Then there is a blue one which is a cationic [acid] stone.

All you have to do is use the opposite ionization of foods and it will dissolve either one of them!

I queried:

What does ionization mean?

Dr. Reams replied:

Ionization [to give a molecule or particle of matter an electric charge], to make it simple is something like silver plating or nickel plating or chromium plating in tanks.

It is either putting something together or taking it apart by electrolysis.

Ionization takes the stones apart. The stones then break down in little particles and pass out of the body system.

How many people who have suffered the agonizing pain of either gallstones or kidney stones would have welcomed this information!

21

THE ROAD THAT LEADS TO STROKES

**Strokes
and the
American
Way of Life**

Medical doctors call strokes: Cerebrovascular Accidents.

I believe that it is more than an "accident." It is a tragedy, much of it brought about by the American way of life, of improper eating, and the competitive, tense society in which we live.

Cerebrovascular accidents are the most frequent cause of brain damage. They are internal accidents arising from a variety of different causes. These impair circulation of blood to the brain.

The brain, more than any other organ, depends heavily upon a rich and continuing supply of oxygen from the blood stream. It has been estimated that the brain receives 25% of the heart's total output of oxygen-rich arterial blood. Yet the brain tissue represents less than one-tenth of the total body weight.

Other organs, including the heart, have some degree of reserve to accommodate temporary interruption.

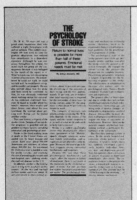

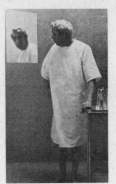

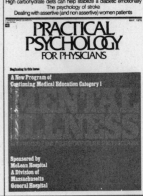
Stroke is the third leading cause of death in the United States, exceeded only by heart disease and cancer. Each year, about 500,000 Americans are stricken, of whom about 200,000 die. An estimated $1.2 billion a year is needed to care for stroke victims—not counting the cost of attending physicians and non-hospital care—making stroke the costliest disease in the U.S.

In addition, stroke is the *leading cause of long-term disability* in this country. Of the two and one-half million stroke survivors, about 30 per cent return to their normal activities, about 55 per cent are capable of carrying on the activities of daily living, and the rest, approximately 15 per cent, are so helpless that total nursing care is required for the remainder of their lives. In stroke victims under 50, the prognosis is that about 80 per cent can return to work.

Stroke is a sudden catastrophic event that dramatically affects every parameter of life. Mobility, speech, thought, retention, sensation, family relationships, and occupation are all affected to some degree. Moreover, the neurological deficit triggers strong emotional mechanisms and responses.

The psychological state of the stroke patient varies with age, personality profile, and how soon after the stroke event the patient is observed. Generally, the younger the stroke victim, the greater the chances are for complete recovery. Pre-existing personality structure is largely responsible for the behavioral responses to the stroke. The effectiveness of rehabilitation therapy also enters into the psychological state. Success breeds confidence. Failure leads to depression and regression.

The brain, however, does not. Any limitation of oxygen supply due to circulatory distress of any kind leads to actual death of the nerve cells within one to four minutes.

A stroke (known also as apoplexy) is the most common of cerebrovascular accidents. This is the destruction of brain tissue due to hemorrhage or rupture of a blood vessel within the brain.

**Thrombosis
A
Clot**

It may also be caused by <u>thrombosis</u>, which is formation of a clot within the brain. This usually comes as a result of severe <u>arteriosclerosis</u>, which is a thickening of the cerebral blood vessels until a blockage occurs.

What happens is that suddenly, without warning, the brain tissue is deprived of its vital oxygen supply. The result may be a degree of neurological loss ranging from (1) a very slight weakness of a few muscle groups on one side of the body, (2) to a paralysis of an entire side of the body, or (3) death. This type of previously mentioned stroke most commonly occurs after the age of 50.

**Embolism
and
Aneurysm**

An <u>embolism</u> (an obstruction of a blood vessel by a foreign particle) usually occurs with young people and children, and is associated with heart disease. An embolism can result from rheumatic heart disease or may be the result of a developmental defect.

Then there is the <u>aneurysm</u> (weak spot in the cerebral blood vessel) which suddenly expands and breaks.

High blood pressure is a complicating factor

of strokes.

Dr. Reams explained:

Everyone has their own blood pressure. There are a lot of people ... for instance, musicians and perfectionists whose blood pressure is always very, very high all their lives. Their blood pressure never gets down low. With others it is very low all the time.

Blood pressures only become dangerous whenever they exceed the limits of that particular individual.

I then asked:

So there's no such thing as a normal blood pressure? Can we arrive at a flat figure and say that this is normal?

Dr. Reams replied:

There is a line in which most people's blood pressure will be found. But we cannot make a flat figure.

I questioned:

Why would musicians have a higher blood pressure?

Dr. Reams answered:

Because musicians are so keyed up. They're as tight as an E string. They've got to be absolutely perfect. Actors, actresses and some ministers are also very keyed up. I have some people whose blood pressure never gets under 200 over 110. This is the way they've been all their life!

I asked:

Doesn't this disturb you then when you take their urinalysis?

Dr. Reams replied:

Not at all, because they have had it all their years.

To determine whether it is in the dangerous level, you have to start with them when they are young and you have to follow it over the years. Their body chemistry would tell me whether they are in a dangerous high blood pressure zone. As long as their blood pressure is normal for them, it does not show up in our tests. However, when it is abnormal for them it does show up.

I then asked him:

My mother, as an example, died from a massive stroke. She was not taking any insulin or orinate. What would have caused this stroke? My parents were from Lebanon.

Dr. Reams suggested:

There could have been too much salt in her system over the years. Or it could have been a lack of potassium in her diet.

Dr. Reams had not studied the diets or diseases peculiar to certain countries. But he did state that the people who have had a great choice in diet are about the same all over the world, as far as health problems are concerned.

22

THE ANSWER FOR ARTHRITIS AND RHEUMATISM

**12
Million
Suffer
in the U.S.**

Many people are confused on the meaning of arthritis and rheumatism.

Arthritis
Inflammation of a joint, and inflammations of structures in the vicinity of a joint.

Rheumatism
This is a term used only by laymen to describe any large number of conditions associated with aches and pains in muscles, tendons and joints.

It is estimated that over 12 million people suffer from these ailments, of which over 1 million are partially or totally disabled.

One popular medical information book published for the general public states:

There is no diet, special food, drug, mechanical contrivance or electrical apparatus that possesses any specific value in the treatment of arthritis.[1]

While this statement appears very official looking, it is the opinion of the author that it is untrue. Diet can often be most effective in the treatment of arthritis.

I asked Dr. Reams:

When a person comes to you and just gives you their name, can you tell just by looking at their chart whether they have arthritis or rheumatism or are prone to get it?

---

[1]Harold T. Hyman, M.D., *The Complete Home Medical Encyclopedia*, New York, Avon Books, 1971, pp. 105-106.

**A
Revealing
Result**

Dr. Reams replied:

Yes, I can. And we have given people diets who have had problems for years and years and years. In fact one of our first patients had acute arthritis for 17 years. He could not turn over in the bed or bathe himself or walk to the bathroom in 6 years. In one week, we had him feeding himself. In two weeks he was able to turn over in the bed and get up in the wheelchair to go to the bathroom. By the third week he was able to drive his own car away from our retreat. His wife brought him here, but he drove it away. He told me:

I'm just as good now as I want to be.

And so he left.

I then asked the Doctor:

What about aspirin and other patent medicine drugs? Do they just treat the symptom and not the cause?

Dr. Reams replied:

Yes, that is true!

Through proper diet, the cause of arthritis and rheumatism can be treated and the individual will respond. We have proved this hundreds and hundreds of times. Of 24,000 people I tested in 1970-71 alone, there were 10,000 that were termed terminally ill by their doctors and during that two years we only lost 5.

Just think of it. There are 12 million people suffering from arthritis-related ailments. Yet very few ever think of looking at diet to relieve them of some, if not all, of the misery this disease imposes on them. Again, Dr. Reams has a track record of success!

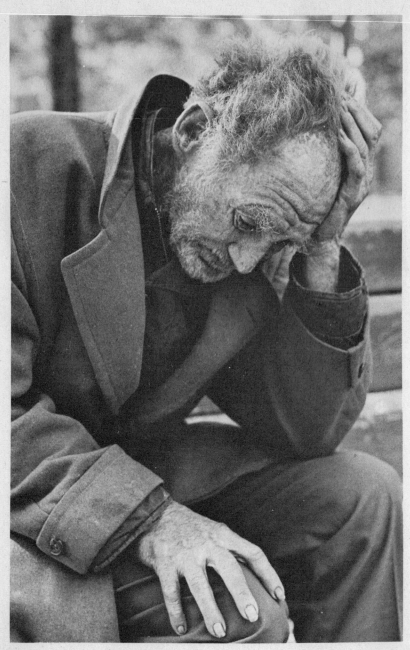

Can we not offer hope through proper nutrition?

April 1976

Hospital Practice

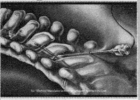

April 1976

Volume 11 Number 4

Hospital Practice

The Management of Obesity
Thaddeus S. Danowski

Preventing Infection in Intravenous Therapy
Dennis G. Maki

IN THE CLINICAL STRATEGY SECTION

Respiratory Infections in Children
Common Complaints of the Elderly

Editor ... Deception in Medicine

... es have risen ... s been no di- ... Longevity has changed little, and the major ill nesses such as malignancy ...

... stitutions discharge many activities simultaneous-ly. Excellence requires that each activity be supe-rior. For instance ...

Nowhere are the consequences of this situation more vivid than in health care for the elderly. Physical consequences of aging are considered medical problems, and sufferers are commonly in-stitutionalized. As a consequence, medical ex-penses for the elderly are three to 11 times those of other population groups. There are few incentives and fewer opportunities for care at home and maintenance of independent function by the eld-erly. They live in dread of being stored in hospitals and nursing homes, their minds blunted by tran-quilizing drugs. It cannot be denied that aging poses special problems in health. It equally cannot be denied that there are effective means of manag-ing these problems which receive scant attention.

Medical schools and centers are the pacesetters in creating the present state of affairs. It is they, not the practitioners, who emphasize technology, employ increasing numbers of drugs and tests in the name of thoroughness without adequate con-trol, and practice institutional medicine virtually without venturing into the community where disease occurs and runs its course.

(continued on page 18)

First, it is not static. In medicine, a field of con-tinuous change, excellence must be reasserted in each new setting. Second, professionals and in-

This editorial is by Dr. Halsted R. Holman, Professor of Medicine, Stanford University School of Medicine, Stanford, Calif.

Here is the medical approach to the problems of arthritis.

1. *Important Note:* This drug is not a simple analgesic. Do not administer casually. Carefully evaluate patients before starting treatment and keep them under close supervision. Obtain a detailed history, and complete physical and laboratory examination (complete hemogram, urinalysis, etc.) before prescribing and at frequent intervals thereafter.

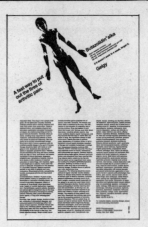

2. Short-term relief of severe symptoms with the smallest possible dosage is the goal of therapy. Dosage should be taken with meals or a full glass of milk.

3. Use lowest effective dosage. Weigh initially unpredictable benefits against potential risk of severe, even fatal, reactions. The disease condition itself is unaltered by the drug.

4. Serious, even fatal, blood dyscrasias, including aplastic anemia, may occur suddenly despite regular hemograms, and may become manifest days or weeks after cessation of drug.

5. Cases of leukemia have been reported in patients with a history of short- and long-term therapy. The majority of these patients were over forty. Remember that arthritic-type pains can be the presenting symptom of leukemia.

6. *Adverse Reactions:* This is a potent drug; its misuse can lead to serious results. Review detailed information before beginning therapy. Ulcerative esophagitis, acute and reactivated gastric and duodenal ulcer with perforation and hemorrhage, ulceration and perforation of large bowel, occult G.I. bleeding with anemia, gastritis, epigastric pain, hematemesis, dyspepsia, nausea, vomiting and diarrhea. abdominal distention, agranulocytosis, aplastic anemia, hemolytic anemia, anemia due to blood loss including occult G.I. bleeding, thrombocytopenia, pancytopenia, leukemia, leukopenia, bone marrow depression, sodium and chloride retention, water retention and edema, plasma dilution, respiratory alkalosis, metabolic acidosis, fatal and nonfatal hepatitis (cholestasis may, or may not be prominent), petechiae, purpura without thrombocytopenia, toxic pruritus, erythema nodosum, erythema multiforme, Stevens-Johnson syndrome, Lyell's syndrome (toxic necrotizing epidermolysis), exfoliative dermatitis, serum sickness, hypersensitivity angiitis (polyarteritis), anaphylactic shock, urticaria, arthralgia, fever, rashes (all allergic reactions require prompt and permanent withdrawal of the drug), proteinuria, hematuria, oliguria, anuria, renal failure with azotemia, glomerulonephritis, acute tubular necrosis, nephrotic syndrome, bilateral renal cortical necrosis, renal stones, ureteral obstruction with uric acid crystals due to uricosuric action of drug, impaired renal function, cardiac decompensation, hypertension, pericarditis, diffuse interstitial myocarditis with muscle necrosis, perivascular granulomata, aggravation of temporal arteritis in patients with polymyalgia rheumatica, optic neuritis, blurred vision, retinal hemorrhage, toxic amblyopia, retinal detachment, hearing loss, hyperglycemia, thyroid hyperplasia, toxic goiter, association of hyperthyroidism and hypothyroidism (causal relationship not established), agitation, confusional states, lethargy; CNS reactions associated with overdosage.

TWO APPROACHES TO THE SAME PROBLEM

An individual woke up one morning with a swelling in her left leg near her ankle. She had a history of varicose veins. The doctors believed the swelling was caused by phlebitis (inflammation of a vein). The area was red and patchy and tender to the touch. Two years prior, she had broken her leg.

She saw Doctor No. 1.		
She waited in the waiting room 1 hour.	Charge:	$10.00
He saw her for 8 minutes.		
He suggested Butazolidin® alka. *		
He also suggested she see her orthopedic physician.		

She saw her orthopedic physician.		
He took an x-ray. This took 5 minutes	Charge:	$28.00
She waited one-half hour . . . then		
saw the physician for 12 minutes	Charge:	$20.00
He confirmed Doctor No. 1's analysis and		
gave her a prescription for Butazolidin®		
alka. * He also told her to stay in bed, keep	Prescription	$ 5.25
her leg elevated, apply warm compresses		
and take Maalox® with the Butazolidin®		
alka. *		$63.25

Instead, she chose to take 1000 units of	Total	
Vitamin C at each meal and 300 units of	Cost	
Vitamin E at each meal . . . and stay on	of	
her feet. **	Vitamins	$ 5.50

Within 2 days the swelling and tenderness disappeared and in 3 days the leg was back to normal. She is also following other natural health habits to eliminate the varicose problem.

  * Butazolidin® alka requires close medical supervision. It can cause very serious side effects. It is a potent drug.

** The above information is for educational data for medical doctors and no one should self-prescribe any form of treatment. It is the opinion of some that the drug recommended would have alleviated the pain but not treated the cause of the problem. Others believe the vitamin and nutrition therapy would correct the cause of the inflammation.

23

THE BRIGHTER SIDE OF DIABETES
AND HYPOGLYCEMIA

**The
Passing
of
Honey**

Of all the serious, chronic diseases that occur in North America and Europe, diabetes is the most prevalent!

We are referring specifically to <u>Diabetes Mellitus.</u>

This medical terminology is from the Greek which in effect means:

The passing of honey.

It is more commonly known as "sugar diabetes."

It has been estimated that two out of every hundred people in the Western world develop diabetes mellitus at some time during their lives. In the United States, some two million Americans have this disease.

A common conception of diabetes is that people develop this from an overindulgence of sweets. This is <u>not</u> true! While the disease can appear at any time, it tends to be more severe the younger the individual is when these symptoms begin.

Diabetes generally results from an insufficient amount of the hormone insulin. These are normally produced by special secreting cells called Beta cells. These Beta cells are located in the islets of Langerhans, which are small clusters of tissue scattered throughout the pancreas. Diabetes is generally detected by sugar in the urine. When the Beta cells fail to function properly a pileup of sugar enters the blood stream.

Revealing Symptoms

Young people especially have symptoms of extreme thirst, extreme hunger, frequency of urination, more copiously than usual. The individual may begin to eat much more than usual, but oddly enough, this steady increase of food intake does not result in any weight gain; rather a steady but gradual weight loss often appears. The person, in a sense, is starving, while their blood retains the sugar.

Itching of the skin, easy exhaustibility, muscular weakness, a fruity odor of the breath, are other symptoms of diabetes.

I asked Dr. Reams:

Have you had cases of diabetes here?

Dr. Reams replied:

Yes, many of them! There are many kinds of diabetes. As an example there is high blood sugar which is hyperglycemia and low blood sugar which is hypoglycemia.

I then remarked to Dr. Reams:

There are some rather exhaustive tests taken in hospitals to determine whether one has hyperglycemia and hypoglycemia. Can you de-

Blindness Linked to Insulin

Rates Turn Higher After Drug's Start

Reston, Va. — (AP) — Researchers say the insulin that has saved millions of diabetics from death may actually cause one of the disease's most ravaging after-effects—blindness.

The first indications that insulin may be a two-edged sword came in results of studies with rhesus monkeys. Test results were announced here yesterday by University of California at Los Angeles researchers.

"The results of our study raise important questions concerning whether insulin, apart from its ability to prolong life, may contribute to the development of diabetic proliferative ocular (eye) disease," said Dr. Alan L. Shabo.

Proliferative diabetic retinopathy is a disease seen in various stages in the majority of diabetics. As it progresses, the disease can result in bleeding inside the eyeball, detached retinas and other complications that can severely hamper vision.

Incidence Rises

In 1930, when animal insulin was not in wide use, new cases of diabetes blindness were less than 1 percent of the national total, he said. But it now accounts for more than 15 percent of new cases.

Among persons with diabetes for more than 11 years figures show the eye disease present in various stages in 64 percent. For those with diabetes for 15 to 20 years, more than 90 percent have eye disease.

Life expectancy for diabetics improved dramatically with insulin therapy, Shabo said, and "it is often asserted that this increased longevity accounts for the increasing incidence" of the eye disease.

The new findings cast doubt on this explanation, he said.

"We believe that the possible role of insulin as a causative factor . . . demands immediate and detailed verification in laboratory and clinical investigations," Shabo said.

10 Million Afflicted

Diabetes is a disease in which the body's ability to burn up sugar is hampered because the pancreas does not produce enough insulin. The condition is controlled through substituting insulin from animals, namely cows, or through weight control and diet.

RPB, a foundation supporting eye research, says statistics show some 10 million Americans have diabetes—half of these cases undiagnosed.

Diabetic eye disease in initial stages is characterized by leaky blood vessels in the eye. Shabo said this could allow leakage of insulin into the eye, which theoretically could be attacked by the eye's defense system to cause or aggravate the disease.

termine their condition simply by a urine/saliva/eye test?

**Going
off
Insulin**

Dr. Reams affirmed his opinion:

Yes! And depending how long they have been on insulin, there are possibilities that we can get them off of it. To some who have been on insulin too long, it has damaged their system whereby our diet cannot help. However, we have had many who have come here who, after proper diet, have been able to go off both injectible and oral insulin.

Dr. Reams never tells anyone not to take insulin or any other medicine prescribed by a physician. Each person must regulate all of his drug intakes himself.

Dr. Reams has had people come to his retreat with a variety of ailments from a bad cold to leprosy . . . and he has witnessed an unusual percentage of success in getting them back on the road to good health via proper diet.

24

THE ANSWER TO CANCER
and the
BRILLIANT SUCCESS WITH LEUKEMIA

**A
Cure
For
Cancer**

Cancer is a disorderly growth of tissue cells . . . according to medical doctors.

Dr. Reams disagrees! Dr. Reams says that this is the reason they have not found the answer for a cure for cancer. They are looking in the wrong place for it!

Medical doctors say that cancer cells can be compared to weeds in a well-kept garden. If the weeds are not eradicated, eventually the entire garden will die.

Not so . . . says Dr. Reams!

Medical doctors also say that there is a greater incidence of cancer in people over 60.

Again Dr. Reams disagrees:

Cancer is premature aging due to a mineral deficiency in our diet. This may occur before a baby is one year old!

The American Cancer Society reports the following statistics:

Breast cancer will strike 89,000 people this year. Of these, 33,000 women will die.

Lung cancer is the leading cause of cancer deaths. It is projected that 84,000 will die this year of lung cancer. Smoking is the leading cause of lung cancer.

More males die of cancer than females. Approximately 205,000 males die of cancer each year. About 170,000 females die annually.

Virtually every organ and tissue in the human body is vulnerable to cancerous growth. Cancer can be classed today as the most dreaded disease.

**Over
1 Million
Suffer**

Right now, about 35 out of every 100 newborn children may be expected to develop cancer at some time during their lives. Presently there are perhaps over 1 million Americans who suffer from cancer.

I asked Dr. Reams:

Have you seen people at this retreat with cancer?

He answered:

Yes, not only have I seen people here with cancer, but I have seen them here in their late stages. There have been people come, just to accompany their husband or wife. They take the urine/saliva test and I have revealed to them they have advanced carcinoma.

Malignant, "bad," signifies growing very rapidly. Benign, "good," means it might still be growing very rapidly but is contained.

I asked:

You refer to a dying cell, what is that called?

Dr. Reams replied:

Carcinoma. And it would be carcinoma if it was malignant. But cancer is a dead cell. The carcinoma cell is a cell that is still trying to function. It could be compared to an old tire. By looking at

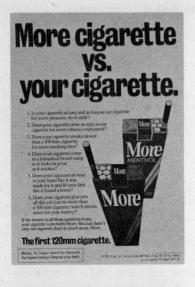

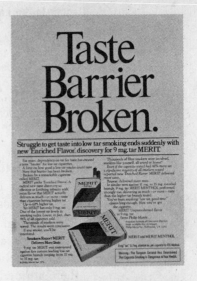

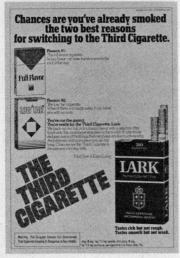

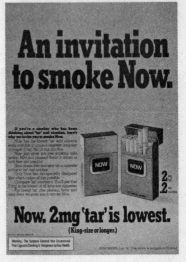

Cigarette ads continue to flourish as does lung cancer!

the urine/saliva charts we can tell whether a person has carcinoma or carcinoma that is probably malignant.

I then questioned:

Suppose a person has been told by his doctor he has 2 to 6 months to live, because of malignant cancer . . . have you had cases like that where the medical profession has given up?

**One Week
To Live
Yet
Still Living**

Dr. Reams replied:

We have had them where they have only had one week to live and they are still living after following our diet!

A dentist, had leukemia which is a type of blood cancer. He was 81 years old and his reserve energy was on the 4 line. I did not think we could keep him living through the night, but we did. He had a lesion about the size of a pea on his lip that would bleed and wound not heal. The medical doctors said he had degenerated arthritis and just had to live with it. In 10 weeks, we were able to send him home with the proper diet and he went back to dental practice! He is the picture of health.

I then asked:

What about leukemia? I know it is a cancer of the white blood cells and that the acute form of leukemia is seen most frequently in children and young people under 15. In fact it kills approximately 1500 young people annually in the United States. A total of 34,000 people, including children, die of leukemia each year. It is a very sad thing when you see children dying of leukemia. Has your urine/sputum analysis been able to detect leukemia and have people responded to your diet?

**Success
With
Leukemia**

Dr. Reams then made some shocking claims:

Yes! We have had children come here with

Environment Blamed For 60% of Cancer

Washington — (UPI) — Between 60 and 90 percent of all cancer stems from enfironmental causes — many of them man-made, Preside... council on Environmenta... said today.

The council's 6th annual r... the incidence of cancer in th... States has more than double... the start of the century, and th... been almost no improvement... vival rates since the 1050s...

ably associated with carcinogenic agents produced by...

...ort:
...m-
...ct
...s
...r-

FOOD

Breakfast Bestseller

Bacon and eggs, toast, waffles, pancakes have their devotees, but the most popular American breakfast is cold cereal with milk.

A Lot of Puff? The competition is hottest in presweetened cereals, which captured 31% of sales last year. Falling sugar prices are encouraging manufacturers to step up introductions of new brands: General Mills is bringing out Fruit Brutes, aiming to win kids away from Kellogg's Fruit Loops, and Ralston Purina is offering Fruity Freakies.

F.D.A CALLED LAX ON CANCER PERIL

House Unit Told of Inaction on Drug Used on Farms

By DAVID BURNHAM

WASHINGTON, March 15— A House subcommittee was told today that more than a decode after the Government was warned that some drugs used to treat billions of chickens, turkeys and swine might cause cancer, has still not removed the drugs from the market.

The target of the criticism was the Food and Drug Administration and its handling of a class of drugs called nitrofurans, widely used on American farms to increase the resistance of poultry and swine to disease and thereby assist in their growth.

...he ...ates ...en- ...ex- ...at

...e Environmental ...n Agency last year found low quantities of cancer agents in the drinking water of all 80 cit... whose supplies it t...

Average American Drank 27 Gallons of Soft Drinks in a Year

Each American drank an average of almost 27 gallons of soft drinks in 1974, according to the National Soft Drink Assn.

The most soft drinks were consumed in the south, the least in the northeast and the northwest, the association said.

Most people eat the wrong foods. Is it any wonder we are sick?

leukemia and we have had 100% success!

I repeat, young people and adults have come here with leukemia and we have had 100% success. I don't know whether we can do that in all cases, but so far, we have had 100% success. Leukemia is one of the easiest things to correct.

The reason this is so easy to correct is because the cause of leukemia is that the body cannot assimilate Vitamin A. If you take Vitamin A by the pound, the body with leukemia will still reject it.

All we do is get the body to accept Vitamin A by various methods with each individual. And it is remarkable how they recover.

I was amazed and remarked:

As a reporter, it seems difficult for me to believe that here you, Dr. Reams, have had 100% success in treating leukemia in children and adults by this, what appears to be a very simple urine/saliva analysis and diet control . . . and yet many in the medical profession in despair do not know how to stop young children from dying with all their drug therapy. And here you have what might be an answer!

Dr. Reams replied:

The amazing thing is that the people who are sent here with leukemia are sent by doctors. And we are able to help them.

You see, we know what a healthy individual's body chemistry should read like. We know those numbers. And we pattern their diet to bring those numbers back to perfect. There are no two individuals alike. And each individual we see, we give a custom-prepared diet.

I asked Dr. Reams:

Why do you say that the loss of reserve energy causes cancer?

CANCER

"All cancer is caused because of a lack of minerals."
Dr. Carey Reams

According to Dr. Carey Reams . . .

Brain Tumor   Lack of POTASSIUM

Lung Cancer   Requires 60 different minerals.
There are more elements by number
than rest of body put together.
Deficiencies in these minerals
lead to cancer.

Breast Cancer   Lack of MANGANESE

Stomach Cancer   Body is too acid too long

**Cancer of
Ovaries, Uterus**   Lack of MANGANESE

Prostate Cancer   Lack of MANGANESE

Colon Cancer   Lack of COPPER, IRON, ZINC

Skin Cancer   Lack of VITAMIN A
closely associated with insulin

**The Answer
on
Cancer**

Dr. Reams gave his opinion:

The loss of reserve energy results in a lack of minerals. ***And all cancer is caused because of a lack of minerals.*** *Cancer* <u>is not</u> *like an animal preying upon you at all! Cancer does not actually grow as such.*

As the minerals becomes more deficient in your system, your body has less resistance and as the resistance decreases the size of the cancer increases.

I then questioned:

I have heard of many cases, some friends of mine, where the doctor operates on someone with cancer . . . and the patient seems to die quicker. Does the cancer spread after surgery?

Dr. Reams replied:

Any lowering of the reserve energy, such as that which can be brought about by surgery, causes an increase of these unfavorable conditions. The reason for this is because it takes resistance to make these minerals available to your system. And when you lower your resistance the cancer increases.

I became more intrigued and asked:

Now then, cancer is dead cells. And if they are dead cells, how can a malignant dead cell affect other cells and make them dead . . . if the cell is already dead?

Dr. Reams answered:

There are two ways to explain it. It is something like a rotten apple in a barrel of good apples. Once the cell dies, funguses or bacteria get into it and aggravate the condition. If you can stop the funguses or bacteria . . . many times the body has enough resistance to heal itself. But if it is not stopped, then the bacteria and funguses aggravate

High Cost of Cancer

In a study of 115 families with cancer patients, the median cost of the illness, based on a median duration of 24 months, was $19,054. The study done by Cancer Care, Inc., New York, N.Y., found that total costs related to the illness ranged from $5,000 to more than $50,000.

The median income of these families was $8,000. Health insurance was "the main source of funds," but family loans, life savings, and sale of personal and other property were required to cover costs.

Hospital and doctor expenses accounted for 63.5 percent of all costs. Other frequently reported costs included drugs, transportation, homemaker services, nursing services, equipment, treatments, and lab tests.

the condition and then is often fatal. Even after we stop the activity of the bacteria and fungus, you must still have the mineral. Many cancers neither have any funguses or bacteria in them.

I then wondered:

In any diet attempting to correct this situation, does that dead cell come back to life or is it sloughed off the body?

Dr. Reams answered:

God is not in the Second Hand Part Business

God never repairs a damaged cell. He is not in the second hand part business. He throws out the dead cell or the carcinoma cell and puts a brand new cell in its place. Every cell in the human adult should be changed about every 6 months. If the cell stays in the body longer than that it becomes a carcinoma cell.

This leads to one very interesting fact. Cancer is only premature aging!

Premature aging is brought about by lack of minerals in our diet especially calciums and phosphates and some potassium. When the answer to cancer is found, we will have the answer to longevity.

It was unbelievable! Here I was speaking to a man who claims that he has had brilliant success through diet in curing cancer . . . a man who flatly states what is the cause of cancer and who claims to have a track record to back up his statements. If he is even partially correct, every medical doctor should be beating a path to his door for the sake of millions of cancer patients who may be needlessly dying an agonizing, premature death!

25

YOU MEAN I CAN EAT HOT PEPPERS!

Hot Peppers and Benzene

While at the Interfaith Christian Church retreat high atop the Blue Ridge mountains of Georgia, and on my special lemon fast, I noticed that the dining room tables had jars of hot peppers on them.

This intrigued me, for I love hot peppers but they never agreed with me and caused indigestion and gas.

I asked Dr. Reams:

Why do you have hot pepper jars on the table? I always thought these were bad for you.

Dr. Reams replied:

Peppers contain benzene. Benzene has a number of benefits. In fact, it supplies the mineral that is most needed in our feet and it also supplies the substance that is next to our bones and keeps our bones and muscles from getting in the way of each other. It keeps them separated.

Also a lack of benzene is the cause of sinus problems and it is a rather advanced deficiency when sinus appears.

You may recall people saying, "Oh, my aching feet." These people have a benzene deficiency.

I further inquired:

What else contains benzene?

Dr. Reams informed me:

Not only do hot peppers contain it but radishes, turnips, etc.

Hot Peppers in the Shoes

It was then that I humorously recalled my wife telling me that when she was a little girl she loved to ice skate on the lake in the Hunting Park section of Philadelphia. On bitter cold days, her mother would sprinkle hot pepper in her shoes to keep her feet warm!

I then asked Dr. Reams:

What are the foods that contain arsenic and why are they good for you?

Dr. Reams answered:

Asparagus and celery. The arsenic in vegetables is in the phosphate form and is not poisonous. In fact it is vital for a strong heart! Our hearts contain a large amount of arsenic compared with the other organs and this is what really makes the heart different from all the other organs.

I then asked Dr. Reams an intriguing question:

Would you say that raw, leafy vegetables are more beneficial than apple pie and ice cream?

Dr. Reams replied:

No, I cannot make a flat statement like that. Everyone has allergies and I couldn't name any

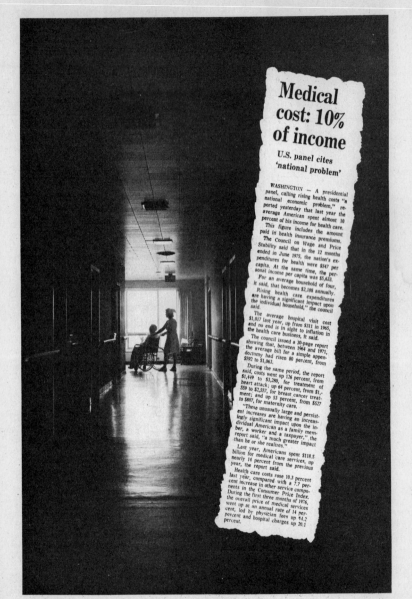

Medical cost: 10% of income

U.S. panel cites 'national problem'

WASHINGTON — A presidential panel, calling rising health costs "a national economic problem," reported yesterday that last year the average American spent almost 10 percent of his income for health care.

This figure includes the amount paid in health insurance premiums.

The Council on Wage and Price Stability said that in the 12 months ended in June 1975, the nation's expenditures for health were $547 per capita. At the same time, the personal income per capita was $5,613.

For an average household of four, it said, that becomes $2,188 annually.

"Rising health care expenditures are having a significant impact upon the individual household," the council said.

The average hospital visit cost $1,017 last year, up from $311 in 1965, and no end is in sight to inflation in the health care business, it said.

The council issued a 30-page report showing that, between 1964 and 1971, the average bill for a simple appendectomy had risen 80 percent, from $592 to $1,063.

During the same period, the report said, costs went up 126 percent, from $1,449 to $3,280, for treatment of heart attack; up 64 percent, from $1,559 to $2,557, for breast cancer treatment; and up 53 percent, from $527 to $807, for maternity care.

"These unusually large and persistent increases are having an increasingly significant impact upon the individual American as a family member, a worker and a taxpayer," the report said, "a much greater impact than he or she realizes."

Last year, Americans spent $118.5 billion for medical care services, up nearly 14 percent from the previous year, the report said.

Health care costs rose 10.3 percent last year, compared with a 7.7 percent increase in other service components in the Consumer Price Index.

During the first three months of 1976, the overall price of medical services went up at an annual rate of 14 percent, led by physician fees up 14.2 percent and hospital charges up 20.1 percent.

food that I could think of that someone would not have an allergy to.

Green, raw leafy vegetables are certainly needed. But the person on low blood sugar may need the apple pie and ice cream. Now that is contrary to all medical practices. But on low blood sugar I break all the rules . . . and they get well!

Perhaps that is why Dr. Reams is so often successful in getting people back on the road to health. He breaks the rules. His belief is, "Why guess when you can be sure." And he goes by the numbers . . . mathematical equations that are precise and which seem to be effective in a great many cases in achieving the end result.

26

TURNING LEMON INTO LEMONADE

Abundant Energy

I am just about at the end of my 3 day fast.

For the last 3 days I have been on a special lemon and distilled water fast. I have had nothing to eat and nothing else to drink.

Multiple thousands before me have taken this same fast. In 1970 and 1971 alone, Dr. Reams tested and designed nutritional programs for over 24,000 people!

Today, on my third day, I have abundant energy. Frankly, I am surprised. I expected to be dragged out and fatigued. Yet I have walked into the dining room at breakfast, lunch and dinner time . . . watched people eating hearty, healthy meals . . . but I have not felt tempted. I would sit down with them and drink my distilled water. That was my meal.

Very few people will believe this. I certainly would not have, for I have never gone on a 3-day fast. The only way one can possibly appreciate and believe the truth of my statements is for them to actually try this method themselves. People have all sorts of opinions about fasts . . . mostly negative. That is because they have never correctly followed one.

Many people think the medical doctor is the end answer to any health problem. They live by their doctor and they will die by their doctor. Many uphold their doctor as a god who can do no wrong, make no wrong diagnosis, prescribe no wrong drug, come up with no wrong answer.

Knowledgeable doctors who are sincere and not led by selfish profit motives will be the first to admit they do not have all the answers to the problems of health.

One day I was visiting some very good friends in Santa Ana, California. They had a lemon tree. It was the first one I had seen, and I couldn't believe they were lemons. They were so big . . . almost as big as an orange. I took one down from the tree and ate the entire lemon. It tasted slightly tart but with a distinctive sweetness. I was amazed . . . for the lemons I had bought in my home supermarkets were always small and very lemony.

Why Not An Orange?

I asked Dr. Reams:

You use the lemon for the fasting period. Why did you pick a lemon as opposed, say, to an orange?

Dr. Reams replied:

The lemon is the only food I know of in the whole world that has a juice that is completely <u>anionic</u>. I am speaking of a fresh lemon, not a reconstituted juice or a canned lemon juice.

By anionic, I mean if you could split one of the molecules wide open and look at it the electrons in orbit would be travelling clockwise.

All other foods are <u>cationic</u> and their electrons are travelling counter-clockwise.

The Perfect Equation

The Equation for perfect health is:

Sugar	pH	Saline	Albumin	Urea
1.5	6.40	6-7C	.04 M	$\frac{3}{3}$
	6.40			

When the entire group of numbers are correlated one with the other, it is possible to calculate exactly where and to what extent disease has entered the body.

Sugar
The normal sugar level is 1.5. If this number is in the 6.0 range it indicates that the individual is a borderline diabetic.

pH
The normal pH level for urine and saliva is 6.40. If the level drops below 6.40 the body cannot utilize Vitamin C. It is important that one's body be brought to the normal pH so there is no energy loss. Continued energy loss eventually ends in major illness. There is no magic diet. A diet must be individualized to meet the mineral deficiencies in your particular body.

Saline
The normal salt level is 6C to 7C. Too much salt is the cause of many heart conditions.

Albumin
The normal level is .04 M. The Albumin count is the number of minute particles in the urine. Urine in a healthy individual (with certain exceptions) should be clear (transparent) when it is voided.

Urea
The normal urea level is 3 over 3, or a total of 6. In this equation, the top reading is the cationic nitrate nitrogen. The bottom reading in the chart above is the anionic ammoniacal nitrogen. If the total of these reaches 20 the heart is overworking and fatigue is evidenced. Crib deaths occur when the urea level reaches around 30. Heart attacks may occur when the two combined numbers total 27 or 28. This part of the equation measures the level of undigested proteins in the body chemistry.

Your Life is in Your Liver

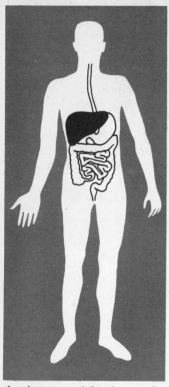

The liver is the largest and perhaps the most complicated organ in the body. It is the most versatile of all organs. Without it the body would perish in 24 hours.

The liver

1. Manufactures bile, an alkaline digestive secretion. This is anionic.

2. Filters old red cells from the blood.

3. Acts as a general detoxifier for the body, removing chemicals and drugs taken in from the outside.

4. Manufactures other complex chemicals needed by the body such as blood proteins, cholesterol and triglycerides.

5. Builds sugar up into a new substance, a special body fuel called glycogen, a complex carbohydrate food material.

The liver normally can survive if only one-quarter of it remained undiseased and functioning. But it is important to remember, that because of this fact, in the destructive disorders of the liver, a great deal of damage can be done before the presence of the trouble is recognized!

The liver has a unique double circulation system. It has an arterial blood supply. It also is involved in the portal blood circulation system. The arterial system returns blood from the liver to the heart. The portal system (which includes the veins containing the absorbed nutriments from the stomach, the duodenum and the small intestine) drain into the large vessel known as the portal vein which passes through a separate network of capillary blood vessels in the liver and then into general circulation again.

Such double circulation makes the liver much more vulnerable to diseases and disorder. Cancer cells, as an example, released from distant sites and carried by the blood stream frequently lodge and grow in the liver.

An improperly functioning liver will not produce its 100% quota of anionic bile to handle the volume of cationic foods that are eaten. Illness occurs. The beginning of illness is the malfunction of the liver. Once the liver is brought back to full functioning power by proper, individualized nutrition, the cause of most illnesses disappear. Your life is in your liver!

So we work the two against each other to get energy. The liver manufactures bile which is an _anionic_ substance with a hydrochloric base. The lemon juice can be converted into millions of different enzymes necessary to maintain life throughout our lives.

It can be converted into these enzymes with less chemical change than any other natural substance known to man. However, there are people who are allergic to lemons.

I asked:

What do you do then?

He replied:

Then we use vegetable juices.

I then queried:

Well, a person's normal diet does not usually include fresh lemons. How does he get this _anionic_ system into his body to develop this energy reserve?

Dr. Reams replied:

Nature can make it from the calciums in our food. Now when the calcium becomes depleted then the liver does not have the substances to manufacture it. When the calciums, and there are over 1/4 million different kinds, mixes with the oxygen, it forms a natural hydrochloric acid.

This lemon/distilled water fast has been very successful in bringing back multiple thousands of people back to perfect health.

Truly, Dr. Carey Reams has found a way to turn a lemon into lemonade!

27

GOOD NEWS FOR OVERWEIGHTS

**We Get
Into A
Rut!**

Socrates said:

Other men live to eat, while I eat to live.

It was Voltaire who observed:

The fate of a nation has often depended upon the good or bad digestion of a prime minister.

How true!

When physical activity begins to decline, many older people put on extra weight. Then with the decline of physical activity, if the body chemistry is not properly functioning, the overall metabolism also begins to slow down.

At this point, too, sometimes the subtle change in our eating habits works adversely.

It is natural for us, being raised in a certain way to like certain foods and all our lives we like to baby ourselves making sure we have the foods that were best to us when we were young . . . so consequently we get into a very, very narrow rut . . . only eating the things we like.

Therefore, many of the glands in our bodies go undernourished.

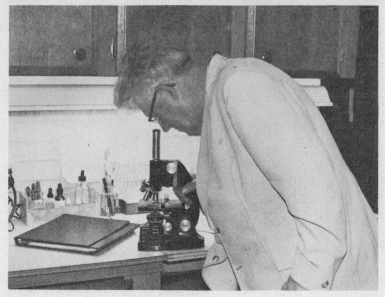

Dr. Carey Reams examining culture in microscope.

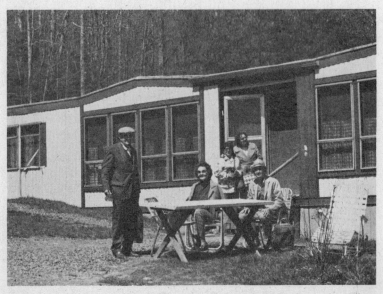

Guests gather at retreat dining hall for a health-planned meal.

Dr. Reams observed:

I have met so many people who have a tongue that is their boss. It tells them what they can eat and what they cannot eat! And those people are the sickest people on earth. They have the lowest energy because anything their tongue rattles for, they hasten to give it to it. So people come through this retreat every week and they say to me . . .

Doctor, how did you know everything I don't like? How did you know?

Well, the very fact is, that the foods they needed most they didn't like, or they wouldn't have been here. In various foods there are various elements.

I then asked Dr. Reams:

I know of one individual who when she takes vitamins . . . she gains weight.

Reasons For Overweight

Dr. Reams replied:

Well, gaining weight is not the worst thing in the world. There are a number of reasons for overweight. One reason is the fact that your liver is not functioning normally. It does not make enough <u>glycogen</u>. The glycogen in the liver goes over to the pancreas. The pancreas makes <u>thyroxin</u> out of it plus some other substances and then it sends it up to the <u>thyroid</u> gland. Then the thyroid gland adds potassium to it which makes old fashioned grandma's soap. That dissolves the excessive oils in our system. And that controls our weight. And one of the reasons we can't put on weight is that it manufactures too much! If it doesn't manufacture enough, then we put on too much weight!

I questioned:

Then the key is in the liver, isn't it?

Dr. Reams affirmed:

Yes, it all goes back to the liver. And you can doctor the thyroid gland until Gabriel blows his

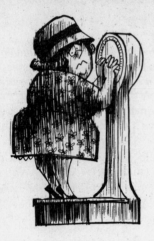

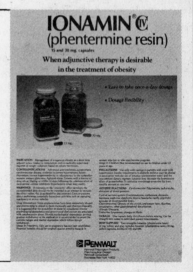

Are drugs the sensible answer to this problem?

trumpet and it won't do any good!

The place to start with a problem like this is with the liver.

But there is another reason for overweight. And that's a lack of calciums in your diet. You become more and more nervous . . . and the more nervous you get the more you eat. The more you eat, the more nervous you get. Therefore it is a neurosis problem because of a calcium deficiency. I don't really believe that there are very many people who are obese . . . less than possibly 2%. These weight clubs treat every person as though they were an obese person and they are not!

I then asked:

**Genetics
and
Overweight**

What about genetics? Do some people inherit overweight problems because of their parents and grandparents?

Dr. Reams replied:

Yes, genetics are another cause of overweight. Many people who have big heads, big feet, big broad shoulders, thick chests and big bones sometimes seek to pattern their body design like the scale they see on those body weight charts. But they should not necessarily try to attain this pattern. You are generally going to look like your ancestors. This is a genetic cause for overweight and there is nothing you can do about it.

I asked:

Are there any more causes for overweight?

Dr. Reams replied:

**Athlete's
Heart**

Yes, there is one more cause for overweight and that is "athlete's heart." This is not a bad thing providing you keep your weight in proportion to the size of your heart. Athlete's heart comes from strenuous exercise when you are young. There are times when one's heart may grow back to normal *but many times it does not.*

If you fail to keep your weight into proportion to the size of your heart, your heart will begin skipping and jumping and begin to give you all kinds of trouble.

Dr. Reams then related an experience:

I had a man come into my office one time that weighed 175 pounds and he looked real thin. But he told me:

> *Dr. Reams, I am nearly dead. I just don't have enough strength to blow my nose.*

He looked in very, very good shape. There was hardly anything wrong with the man. After I examined his urine the equation numbers were almost perfect. I asked him if he lost any weight in the last 3 months. He said he had lost 25 pounds. I asked him why he did this. He said:

> *My family was afraid I was going to have a heart attack and I was about starving myself to death.*

I told him to put that weight back on because his heart was oversized. He had worked hard when he was young and developed "athlete's heart." It was important that he keep his weight in proportion to the size of his heart. When he followed my advice, put the weight back on, he was a different man completely.

Don't try to be like the scale . . . be yourself! If your overweight is by genetics, be satisfied the way God made you. If you follow the rules of good health your weight will stay where it is supposed to be.

It is Dr. Reams' opinion that overweight is not a *cause* for heart attacks. See page 78 for the chapter on heart attacks and their cause and page 166.

28

THE RIGHT AND WRONG WAY TO BATHE

**90%
of All
Operations
Can Be
Avoided**

It is Dr. Reams personal opinion that over 90% of all operations can be avoided!

I reminded him that if this were followed the hospitals would either have to go out of business or advertise for patients. Of course, there is no money in good health!

I read that in Old China a doctor was paid as long as his patient kept well. His payment stopped when the patient got sick. To this Dr. Reams reminded me:

And many times he was beheaded if the patient died!

Of course, I would not advocate that in America, but we should certainly start paying more attention to the cause of disease and not be so concerned with treating symptoms.

It was Jonathan Swift who wrote:

The best doctors in the world are Doctor Diet, Doctor Quiet and Doctor Merriman.

When I was going to school in Girard College in Philadelphia we were required to take a shower every night. Girard College is a grammar and high school for fatherless boys.

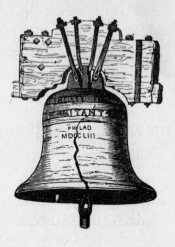

The Constitution of this Republic
should make special provision
for MEDICAL SCIENCE.
To restrict the art of healing
to one class
will constitute
the bastile of Medical Science.
All such laws
are un-American
and despotic.

Benjamin Rush, Physician
Signer of the
Declaration of Independence

By the time I graduated after 10 years stay, I got rather tired of bathing every night. I asked Dr. Reams:

I hear you believe that Americans use too much soap.

Dr. Reams replied:

Bathe without Soap

Yes, I do advocate a bath every day but not soap every day; in fact, not very often. Soap takes the oil off your skin of which nature puts on there to keep Vitamin C into your system. If you take that oil off, then the Vitamin C escapes and you have a cold all the time, especially in the winter.

One of the worst times in the world to use soap is at the first sign of spring. So many people get pneumonia then. Their blood is thick and starts to thin and their body chemistry is making a slight change ... they lose their Vitamin C and consequently have problems.

I then questioned:

Well, if you don't use soap, how do you take a bath?

Dr. Reams answered:

If you must use soap, then take it in the shower and wash. Then put water in the tub with oil and lie in the oil for 10 or 15 minutes. Or a sauna after a bath will produce a little perspiration to put the oil back on but don't use soap again or you will wash it off. Just rinse it off.

I was reminded of what Mark Twain said in 1900:

Soap and education are not as sudden as a massacre, but they are more deadly in the long run.

Well, I couldn't get out of taking a bath nightly, but at least I won't have to use soap!

29

THE MISINFORMATION ON MENOPAUSE

The Truth About Menopause

Menopause is a problem which is often discussed in popular journals as well as medical journals; menopause for men as well as menopause for women.

It was Bob Hope who said:

Middle age is when your age starts to show around your middle.

And Diane De Poitiers who observed:

The years that a woman subtracts from her age are not lost. They are added to the ages of other women.

Menopause is often thought of occurring during the middle years of life. I asked Dr. Reams:

What is menopause?

He replied:

In order to understand menopause you must start with the boy and girl when they are born. Each will use the same amount of calciums until the young lady comes into young womanhood or full puberty. At that time she will use 700 times more calciums per day than a normal man.

This will continue throughout her entire productive-bearing age. The only thing that will cause her to go out of the productive age is that nature has so made us and controls us by the timing of our glands, that at a certain age the calciums will drop below normal, causing the menstrual period to cease. This occurs at the end of the productive bearing age which generally takes place in the 40's or 50's but sometimes even later than that. In the case of Sarah in the Old Testament, she was 90 years old when Isaac was born.

How Menopause Begins

However, anytime the calciums drop too low, at any age, 13, 15, 20, 30 or 40 or any age, then it brings the menopause into existence. And if it lasts long enough it will affect the menstrual flow and cause many kinds of complications. When this occurs the individual becomes more nervous. To that individual the entire world is dropping out from under them. They are difficult to live with. They are angry but not fighting people; rather fighting for their whole life.

I asked Dr. Reams:

Would you say that such a condition is the reason for many divorces today?

Dr. Reams replied:

Yes, many couples are getting divorces after they have been married 20 or 30 years. This is because the calciums are too low in their diet. They still love each other but the low calciums make them so irritable that they just cannot stand each other.

This has become a concern of psychologists and psychiatrists all over the world.

I wondered about vitamins in this role and asked Dr. Reams:

Can this lack of calcium be corrected by people simply running out and taking calcium pills?

Dr. Reams answered:

No, that is not the answer! There are more than 1/4

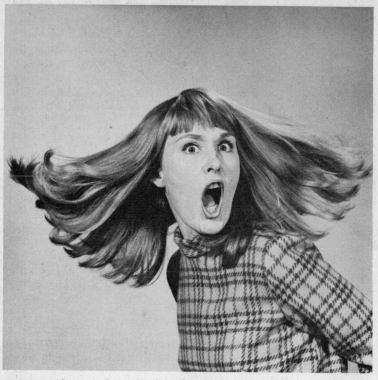

Are many divorces brought about by poor nutrition? Do you sometimes
feel like the individual pictured above?

million different calciums and you must take the right kind of calcium. These 1/4 million different kinds of calciums can be divided into 7 different classes.

I questioned Dr. Reams further:

What about men? Do they also get menopause?

Men and Menopause

Dr. Reams replied:

When men's calciums get too low, they also become nervous and excitable just like women. It is not something which is just peculiar to women. However, it appears only to count when women get nervous.

The symptom of menopausal men and women is most frequently evidenced by nervous tension brought about, of course, by calcium deficiency.

And this can occur at any age. If the calcium drops below a certain level the menstrual flow will stop forever. It is nothing unusual to find girls under 20 years of age who have already ceased their menstrual cycle for life. Many times girls never come into puberty because their calciums are not high enough. There can be, of course, other genetic reasons but calciums are one important reason.

Use of Estrogen Questioned

Dr. Reams does not believe there is a genuine reason for giving estrogen unless the ovaries have been removed or have become so damaged by carcinoma or cancer that they cannot function. This is usually because they do not have enough manganese in their diet. Manganese is one of the elements of life and without manganese there would be no life of any kind upon this planet.

I asked Dr. Reams:

Now you said that during child-bearing days, a woman requires 700 times more calciums than men. How does she achieve this daily quota intake?

Dr. Reams replied:

Well, it should be in your food but our foods today are so depleted in calciums. Cramps, as an example, are caused by a calcium deficiency. This is why women experience cramps during their menstrual period. It is because their body is telling them they are deficient in calcium.

I further questioned Dr. Reams:

If you say that a woman needs more calcium, in what foods can she get it?

Dr. Reams answered:

This is difficult to answer because of the calcium deficiency of most foods grown in the United States. I would recommend that for the highest calciums content, a housewife buy fruits and vegetables grown in the western states, such as California, Arizona, Washington and Oregon. A urine/saliva test and a balanced calciums supplement would be beneficial.

Millions of women throughout the world suffer needlessly each month by menstrual cramps because they do not listen to the monthly message their body is telling them. Yet the answer is so simple that it would almost appear unbelievable. Yet truth is stranger than fiction.

30

THE BLIND SHALL SEE . . .
NEW HOPE FOR GLAUCOMA AND CATARACTS

**The
Tragedy
of
Glaucoma**

Glaucoma afflicts 3% of all people over 60 years of age. It, however, is not limited to the elderly.

Glaucoma is a disease in which the pressure within the eyeball is increased. If this increased tension becomes great enough, it can lead to irreparable damage to the eye. The result is blindness.

The underlying cause of glaucoma is unknown to the medical profession.

What occurs is that (sometimes rapidly, sometimes gradually) there is an increase in the fluid tension inside the eye. This is due to the formation of more intraocular fluid than is able to escape through the tiny canals which normally drain it from the eye and maintain a constant pressure balance within the eyeball.

The tragedy of glaucoma is that it can be detected very early in the disease stage by a painless, simple, and accurate procedure used in the doctor's office. A pressure-measuring instrument is used called a <u>tonometer</u>.

One of the early symptoms of glaucoma is the appearance of halos around lights. There may also be pain and a sense of fullness in the eyeball.

Glaucoma usually develops in one eye and if untreated, will affect the other eye.

Acute glaucoma is evidenced by a sudden onset of pain in the eye, headache, marked reduction in vision, nausea and vomiting, and dilatation of the pupil. When this occurs, surgery is often advised to save the sight. This surgery is called an <u>iridectomy</u>. A piece of the iris is removed in order to permit fluid to escape from the anterior chamber of the eye. If surgery is performed quickly (within a few hours before loss of vision) it is usually successful.

A Better Answer

But I believe <u>prevention</u> and <u>proper diet</u> provide a better answer.

Dr. Carey Reams believes that glaucoma is also a result of Vitamin A deficiency in the system.

I asked Dr. Reams to explain this.

It is another form of anemia—or another form of leukemia. Leukemia is a Vitamin A deficiency and is a type of anemia.

However, let me make something real clear. There are no two cases of anemia or Leukemia alike. Everyone of them present different problems and sometimes they are very difficult to zero in on to discover the actual cause of the lack of Vitamin A.

I questioned:

Have you consulted with different people who have had glaucoma and taken tests on them?

Dr. Reams replied:

Yes, many. We have not only had glaucoma . . . but we have had cataracts to disappear. A cataract is a partial or complete opacity of the crystalline lens or its capsule.

And we have seen both glaucoma and cataracts disappear just by diet alone! The individual's vision comes back to normal.

However, if a person has been on insulin for many years, and the muscles of the eyeball, especially to the retina of the eye, are badly damaged . . . and the muscles are damaged to where the brain waves cannot go into the eye . . . sometimes that is irreparable . . . except by a miracle of God. And I have seen God work miracles also!

It was then I remembered when Jesus Christ was followed by a great multitude when two blind men by the side of the road called out: "Have mercy on us, O Lord, thou son of David" (Matthew 20:30-34). The crowd rebuked the blind men for stopping Christ. The Bible tells us:

Jesus had compassion on them, and touched their eyes; and immediately their eyes received sight, and they followed Him.

(Matthew 20:34)

The one attribute I admire most of Dr. Carey Reams is his humble compassion for the sick and his dedication to attempting to bring them back on the road to recovery through diet.

NEW HOPE FOR BREAST CANCER

The Phantom of the Night!

Perhaps of any illness, the one most dreaded by women is breast cancer! It is the phantom of the night suddenly striking unexpectedly and changing her whole life pattern.

It evidences itself in major mutilating surgery that in part "de-womanizes" a woman and requires a lengthly period of readjustment to life. For women, it is a fear beyond all fears. And this deadly disease is no respecter of persons. It strikes at all strata of society from motion picture stars and those high in government circles to the humble mother on welfare.

The medical approach to breast cancer is as follows:

1. *Radical Mastectomy*
   When there is no evidence of peripheral spread (or, at the most, signs of minimal involvement of the axillary lymph glands on the affected side), the treatment of choice, medically, is radical mastectomy—removal of the involved breast, the underlying pectoral muscles, and the contents of the ipsilaterla axilla. Even in the best of circumstances, 10-year survival rates of 50% are

unusual. Moreover, even when these "clinical cure rates" approach or surpass 50%, the disease may recur with fatal outcome as late as 20 years after surgery.[1]

2. Simple Mastectomy

Some specialists prefer simple mastectomy followed by radiotherapy as the primary treatment of choice, if the malignancy is confined to the breast without spread to the adjacent muscles or to the regional nodes or beyond. The difficulty is in the determining if the cancer has spread to other parts of the body. Many physicians believe the simple mastectomy leaves much to be desired.

3. Radiotherapy

Radiotherapy is usually given after an operation. When the cancer has travelled from its original site in the breast to other internal organs, radiotherapy is considered of little value.

The efficacy of postoperative irradiation in improving survival or recurrence rates has not been demonstrated.[2]

4. Chemotherapy

Complications, which may follow the use of any chemotherapy agent, are steadily increasing in frequency.[3] Chemotherapy is the treatment of infections by use of chemicals. Nausea, vomiting, diarrhea and temporary loss of hair are some of the side effects of chemotherapy treatment. The "cure rate" with chemotherapy leaves much to be desired. Its side effects can be devastating.

---

[1]David N. Holvey, M.D., *The Merck Manual of Diagnosis and Therapy* (Rahway, N.J.: Merck Sharp & Dohme Research Laboratories), 1976, p. 876.

[2]Marcus A. Krupp, M.D., *Current Medical Diagnosis & Treatment* (Los Altos, California: Lange Medical Publications), 1976, p. 405.

[3]*Ibid.*, p. 409.

DRUGS IN THE CANCER WAR

...They assume a larger role

By Patrick Young

FROM ST. PETERSBURG BEACH, FLA.

Cancer chemotherapy is coming into its own.

Twenty years ago about one patient in four could expect to live free of the disease for five years or more; today that figure is one in three. And the use of anticancer drugs is credited with making much of the difference.

It has not been an easy achievement, however, nor an assured one.

To Your Health

Cancer still kills; two-thirds of its victims die in less than five years. "You cannot treat anybody with anything and guarantee a cure for cancer," says Dr. Nicholas Bottiglieri, an American Cancer Society vice president. Yet Bottiglieri and others see an ever brighter future for anticancer drugs.

"I have never been as excited in 35 years of medicine as I am today about the potential of chemotherapy in combination with surgery and radiation," he says.

'The Drugs Can Clean Up'

The importance of drugs in combination with surgery and/or radiation treatments is one that has evolved only in recent years. But it is one that is winning increasing recognition and acceptance.

Surgery and radiation are essentially local treatments and ineffective if the primary cancer has metastasized—or spread—as have up to 75 per cent of all cancers by the time of diagnosis. Drugs alone, on the other hand, do not work well against large, solid tumors, the kinds that characterize breast and lung cancers.

So, says Dr. Ralph Johnson, chief of radiation oncology at the National Cancer Institute (NCI), "the surgeon or radiation therapist must reduce the tumor bulk so the drugs can clean up."

The twin realizations that cancer has often spread before it is first detected and that drugs can kill off tiny tumors has led to a major shift in chemotherapy. Increasingly, physicians are giving drugs to patients as soon as the cancer is found rather than waiting to see if the cancer reappears after surgery or radiation.

Surgery and radiation appear to have largely reached their limits in cancer therapy. So now the emphasis is on chemotherapy in combination with the older treatments. But while together they may increasingly prolong and save lives, the battle against malignancy remains a difficult one. Scientists foresee no magic potion that will quickly cure cancer.

With these statistics, is there a better way than drugs and surgery?

**33,000
Die
Annually**

The American Cancer Society reports that each year about 89,000 women are diagnosed as having breast cancer. And of this number, 33,000 die annually. When the cancer in the breast has spread to the surrounding nodes, the survival rate is only 56% over a 5-year period.

I asked Dr. Reams about these breast cancer operations and his opinion on them.

Dr. Reams informed me:

It is well worthwhile to first try the proper diet and not be too hasty about an operation.

However, sometimes breast cancer starts with a malfunction of the central nervous system which does not go through the spinal column but goes down through the side of the neck. It has a branch in the central nervous system that goes through each breast and also goes to the heart and to the lungs, the stomach, the pancreas and to the complete sexual organs.

If there is damage to that branch of the nerve that goes to the breast, then surgery is essential.

There is another branch from this central nervous system that is also slightly intermingled with the glands of the body. It is like the links of a chain . . . anything that affects one affects the other. Therefore even if you discover that the breast nerve has been damaged; then the diet does get the body in shape to withstand the operation with a lot less suffering.

**One Breast
May Involve
The Other**

I then asked Dr. Reams:

If a woman develops cancer in one breast is it most likely also to develop in the other breast?

Dr. Reams suggested:

You seldom ever find one breast involved without

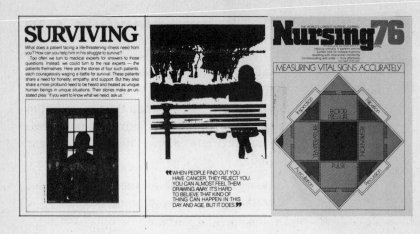

> WHEN PEOPLE FIND OUT YOU HAVE CANCER, THEY REJECT YOU. YOU CAN ALMOST FEEL THEM DRAWING AWAY. IT'S HARD TO BELIEVE THAT KIND OF THING CAN HAPPEN IN THIS DAY AND AGE, BUT IT DOES.

Evelyn Bourgault Antil, RN, MS, former inservice instructor at Burbank Hospital, Fitchburg, Mass., discovered that she had breast cancer in 1972, just one year after becoming Service Committee Chairman with the Massachusetts Cancer Society. After a radical mastectomy, she returned to work, only to discover a lump in her other breast in 1974. The second breast changes were treated with chemotherapy and cobalt treatments. In 1975, she returned with widespread metastases.

At the time of this interview, Mrs. Antil was on chemotherapy. That treatment, the last available to her, failed. On February 24, 1976, Evelyn Bourgault Antil died.

'After the test results came back, my doctor told me I'd have to have a biopsy. He said, though, that "Nine times out of ten these things are benign." And his secretary said the same thing. In fact, everyone did. They were very careful to avoid that dread word—cancer. I knew why—because they truly hoped I didn't have it, because they wanted to encourage me.

'Before the first biopsy, I signed the papers saying the doctors could do whatever was necessary. I knew that could mean a mastectomy if the biopsy was positive.

'When I woke up after surgery, the sense of the missing breast wasn't as alarming as seeing that Thiotepa had been added to my I.V. To me that said, "Cancer and spread." Because I knew that Thiotepa was one of those drugs they use in case any cancerous cells have escaped into the bloodstream during surgery. I think that's when my dread of I.V.s started. It wasn't the I.V. itself but rather its significance.

Should more emphasis be placed on chemotherapy research or in nutrition research? Which approach would you prefer to be used on your body?

the other! And usually it also involves the ovaries, the uterus and the vagina area to some degree. So the very first thing one should do is work on a diet to try to replace into the system the deficient elements necessary to restore that organ or organs to normal.

I questioned Dr. Reams:

If there is any one mineral that is of greatest benefit in the prevention of breast cancer, what mineral would that be?

The Power of Manganese

Dr. Reams replied:

Manganese! Manganese has the power within itself to leave offspring. Manganese is a very essential element to the reproduction organs in both male and female. Manganese is becoming more and more deficient in our foods. It can only be made available to our system in phosphated manganese form.

Dr. Reams believes that where possible every other available method of correcting breast cancer should be used first. An individualized diet is of extreme importance to replace the minerals one's body is deficient in. Surgery should only be considered as the last resort!

I asked Dr. Reams:

What are some of the symptoms that may indicate there is cancer in the breast?

Dr. Reams answered:

One symptom is when the breast begins to feel like little cords inside or like feeling like a ball of twine that has been put into a balloon and blown up; this is one of the first signs of adhesions forming in the nerves of the breast. This is the time to begin working on correcting this situation by body-chemistry analysis and proper diet recommendations.

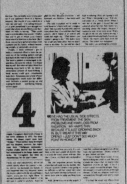

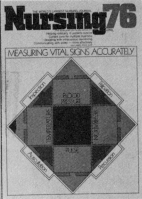

'One afternoon I was sitting in the examination room waiting for my doctor, when a new doctor — a woman doctor — came striding in with my chart. She'd never seen me before, you understand; I have a regular doctor. But she studied my chart for a few minutes and then said to me, "Do you know why you're here?" I said, yes, of course I did — I had a brain tumor that the doctors wanted to examine for possible surgery. I said that they'd looked at it and found it was small, so they weren't going to operate.

'"Well," she snapped, "yes, you have a brain tumor. But it isn't small; it's deep and very large." And she walked out.

'Naturally I was terribly upset. In fact, I was shaking by the time my own doctor finally arrived. When I told him about it, he said to just ignore the other doctor. He said she didn't know my particular case the way he did, that he was the only one qualified to talk about it.

'Finally, at my next clinic appointment, I got up enough nerve to ask my doctor if that was true. He said, "Look, each patient reacts differently to this disease. You're an individual case. Knowing your case and reading about this disease is *our* job. It isn't *your* job. Your job is to be the patient and to let us help you."

'Well, ever since then I haven't read any more cancer articles, unless I can tell from the headlines that they're going to be optimistic. Otherwise, I know I'll just get depressed. If I want to know anything, I ask someone — usually a doctor, but sometimes the nurses, especially if the doctor's busy. If the nurses know, they generally tell me. But if not, they'll tell me to ask my doctor.

If this condition is allowed to continue, then an adhesion forms. The tissue becomes swollen. Then you are said to have carcinoma of the breast.

I next asked Dr. Reams:

Can you actually tell after a woman has had a urine/saliva test if she has breast cancer?

Dr. Reams replied:

We can tell if there are carcinoma cells in the breast by urine tests. And we can tell if it is wide-spread. This should be corrected by diet recommendations.

A breast should be as soft as a wet sponge.

Without Physical Examination

The most unusual aspect of Dr. Reams' claim to spot carcinoma in the breasts is that he does this without any physical examination of the woman or her breast! He simply runs a special urine/saliva test. The individual comes into his library, hands Dr. Reams her laboratory sheet which has the analysis equation on it. Dr. Reams simply verifies that this is her sheet and then proceeds to read to her his analysis. For the individual . . . it is as simple as that. No question is asked of her symptoms. There is no disrobing.

I then asked Dr. Reams:

Have you had women come here to your retreat, for some other reason perhaps, took the test, and you indicated to them that they had carcinoma in their breasts?

Dr. Reams affirmed,

Yes.

No Operation Needed

I further asked:

Have you had people come to this retreat whose doctors said that they had a malignant cancer in their breast and needed an operation who came here, were put on a fast, and a special diet, and then did not need that operation?

Dr. Reams claimed:

Yes, many times. In fact this happened just this last week while you were here. This is a very frequent occurrence. In fact, our success is above 95% or 96%!

I then asked:

What about women with cysts? Is this common in the breasts of women?

Dr. Reams answered:

Yes, there are also fatty tumors in the breast. Fatty tumors are caused because of a trichinosis bacteria that they get from eating pork.

Cysts, many times, are indicated by a watery substance that is different from cancer but in the same category. It is possible for a cyst to develop into a cancer.

Proper nutrition, individually designed for that person, is then indicated.

I have often seen women who have had a breast remove suffer from what appears to be a common aftermath. Their arm swells up sometimes two to three times its normal size. I asked Dr. Reams to amplify on this. He remarked:

When this happens there has been damage then to the central nerve that leads to the breast in that area. There is again where the tangled chain of nerves are affected. In that case, it was necessary to remove the breast. Diet cannot correct this condition. When the nerve is damaged and the messages cannot go through from the brain either through the spinal column or through the central nerve area, which governs the blood flow in that area, then all the cells become carcinoma.

If there is not damage to the nerves, then by diet the swelling can come down.

I then asked Dr. Reams:

You mentioned Manganese as an essential element in the prevention of cancer. Is there any particular food that is rich in Manganese?

Foods Rich in Manganese

Dr. Reams replied:

Any food having seeds is rich in Manganese; that is, seeds you would normally eat. Such foods would include cucumbers, squash, tomatoes and bell peppers.

The reason there is breast cancer is because of a Manganese deficiency. Cancer of the foot is a Benzene deficiency. Cancer of the liver is an Iron and Iodine deficiency, etc. Brain cancer indicates a Potassium deficiency.

So many people try to get these elements into their body in too concentrated a form. And in a strongly concentrated form, the body rebels against it. By proper diet, individualized to that person, these elements can enter the body naturally so that the body accepts them.

I then observed:

Generally after breast cancer, chemotherapy or radiotherapy is used. I guess the purpose of this is to attempt to stop the spread of these cells. Do you agree with this type of therapy?

The Wrong Approach to Breast Cancer

Dr. Reams stated his own frank feelings:

I do not agree with that type of therapy whatsoever. This approach does not replace the nutrients necessary for nature to restore itself. It is only a patched-up affair which may delay death and bring on a death of agony. I have witnessed this so many times.

And then, when a person submits to

New Device Infuses Cancer Outpatients

HOUSTON—Leukemia and other cancer patients at M. D. Anderson Hospital here have been receiving continuous infusions of chemotherapeutic drugs while they go about their usual lives as outpatients. Their medication is administered automatically by a self-contained pump, loaded daily with a drug-filled cartridge and worn strapped to the arm.

"The concept is brilliant," says Dr. Emil J. Freireich, chairman of the department of developmental therapeutics at the hospital. Dr. Freireich calls the liquid infusion system, or LIS, "the best technical approach I've seen to the need for a delicately controlled drug delivery system for the cancer patient undergoing chemotherapy. The LIS has important technical, economic, and psychological advantages over traditional IV drug delivery."

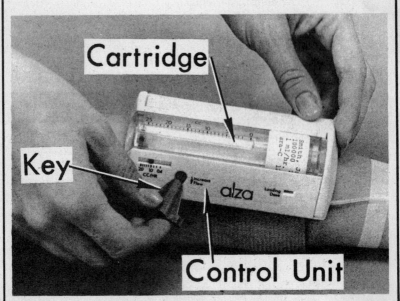

A key is used to set the flow rate of Alza Corp.'s liquid infusion system, which weighs 100 gm, is about the size of a king-sized pack of cigarettes, and can be worn on the arm concealed by a sleeve.

chemotherapy or radiotherapy, it only gets the patient to a place where corrective diet will not have any affect on his body.

Chemotherapy damages the liver, and often causes the hair to fall out. The individual may not die of cancer but they will die of a liver problem. Their livers swell to such an extent that the women look like they are pregnant.

I asked:

If this is true, what do you think of chemotherapy?

Dr. Reams quickly replied:

It is a practice that should be brought to an end.

I then questioned:

You stated that if a woman has cancer in one breast and has it removed, it is quite possible that she may also develop it in the other breast. Is that correct?

Dr. Reams answered:

Yes, your statement is correct, because they are removing the cancer in one tumorous area without removing the cause. But the doctor does not work on the cause of why that cancer was there!

All cancers and all maladies and all diseases are brought about because of a mineral deficiency . . . even those that are aggravated by funguses and viruses.

Breast cancer is caused by a Manganese deficiency!

Cancer Can Be Predicted

I asked Dr. Reams:

With your urine/saliva test, can you predict when and if cancer is going to strike?

Dr. Reams replied:

Yes, with these tests this is possible. We can pre-

dict a few years in advance where cancer is going to strike!

These tests should even be done on children. Whenever you find children whose body cannot assimilate certain vitamins and certain minerals, then you know where the cancer is going to strike even years in advance.

My interest was aroused and I asked:

Do you mean a female child of 12 years of age who takes your urine/saliva test . . . do you think that you can tell whether she will develop cancer in her 20's or 30's or 40's?

Dr. Reams replied:

Yes! If that individual did nothing to correct that diet and we took tests every few months, we could pretty well predict the year that cancer would strike . . . up to 10 years in advance of the actual occurrence!

But prevention should start immediately. No one should wait till the symptoms become evident. Prevention is far, far better than treatment. An ounce of prevention certainly is worth a pound of cure!

The Alternative to Chemotherapy

I asked Dr. Reams:

Now let us suppose that the woman already has had her breast removed and the doctor wishes to place her on a treatment of chemotherapy or radiotherapy . . . what is the alternative for her?

Dr. Reams claimed:

If the breast is removed and then he recommends chemotherapy or cobalt, it simply means the doctor fears that he has not gotten it all and that he may believe that the patient has less than five years to live.

There is an alternative!

We have had many women who after breast re-

moval, refuse to submit to chemotherapy or cobalt. We give them a urine/saliva test. And 95% of those who come have their body respond and they get well.

I am bitterly opposed to anything that will make a patient worse. In my opinion, cobalt and chemotherapy does! It does not solve anything. It has never solved anything.

I wonder how many women, who after reading this, will still not seek the more conservative alternative of having a urine/saliva test and then follow an individualized diet to correct their health problem?

In my opinion the answer is so clear on the side of at least trying proper nutrition first as a preventitive that there is no alternative. Then too, the results of Dr. Reams speaks for themselves!

32

HOW TO FEEL LIKE 21 AT 51

Understanding Urea

Dr. Reams is always available to those at his Georgia retreat. At mealtimes he stops in the dining room, chats with the guests. Early in the morning he stops in their rooms to see how they are faring on the lemon and distilled water fast.

And they have many questions to ask him both on proper nutrition and diet.

One question often asked is:

What is urea?

Dr. Reams answers:

Urea is two different forms of nitrogen . . . nitrate nitrogen and ammonical nitrogen.

Urea, as defined in the Reams test analysis, is undigested protein. The base of proteins is nitrogen and in order to convert the nitrogen to proteins Dr. Reams multiplies the nitrogen by 6.4.

Dr. Reams explains:

In the system, when the body does not properly digest the proteins in turning them into energy, then it forms the urea salt. This urea salt overstimulates the heart causing it to beat much harder each time.

I questioned:

What are the signs of too much urea salt?

**Signs to
Look For**

Dr. Reams suggested:

The signs are fatigue, tiredness, tension. Little molehills become mountains to that individual. Also this is the direct cause of all pectoris heart attacks!

I then asked:

Can a person looking at his urine tell whether he has urea in there or not?

Dr. Reams answered:

No!

On the scale, when Dr. Reams gives a urine/saliva test, he assigns a number on that analytical report. If the individual has a high urea count and a high sugar, it can be brought down within a 24-hour period with proper intake of distilled water.

Dr. Reams further amplified:

If a person has a low blood sugar, you really have a problem on your hands . . . because if you start to bring the urea down by drinking distilled water, you can have a person in a coma very easily. Each person needs an individual approach to their problem.

**Urine
Should Be
Transparent!**

I asked Dr. Reams:

In the medical textbook that I have been reading it says that one's urine should have an amber or straw color. Do you agree with that statement?

Dr. Reams replied:

Only if you drank coffee or have eaten some kind of food with dye in it, or taken some vitamins.

If you are perfectly healthy the urine should be as transparent as the water you drink.

That was an unusual statement. Most people who would take the time to examine the color of their urine would find it a yellow or dark amber. A urine which is not transparent like water could indicate a malfunction in their body. (The exception being as stated previously if they drank coffee or some food with dye or ingested a drug such as some of the sulfa drugs given for cystitis, etc.)

Regular and Decaffinated Coffee

In a previous interview Dr. Reams had made some interesting observations on coffee and I asked him his opinion on the difference between drinking regular coffee and decaffinated coffee. His opinion, as usual, was startling!

Most of the time decaffinated coffee is worse than the regular coffee, because of the preservatives in its manufacture. And what little caffeine is in it is stagnant. Actually, there is less damage in drinking a good fresh coffee than there is in the decaffinated coffees.

Most Americans do not drink enough water and hardly any Americans drink solely distilled water. Because urea causes many health problems I asked Dr. Reams if people should not be drinking more distilled water.

Yes, drinking distilled water would help alleviate this problem of pectoris heart attack.

Extreme fatigue, nervous tension, wrinkles in the forehead . . . all will be alleviated from the drinking of distilled water.

Whenever a doctor puts his stethescope on the heart and if one has a high urea count . . . that heart sounds like a drum. You can hear the heart beating very hard. And you often hear doctors say:

You have a heart as strong as a horse.

All they are really saying is that you have a high urea level and you are in the zone for a pectoris heart attack!

I asked Dr. Reams:

What about the urine tests that are conducted in hospitals and other laboratories?

Dr. Reams replied:

These tests do not differentiate between the soluble urea and insoluable. The tests that I have given are not, to my knowledge, done in any hospital. The urea in the blood changes every few minutes . . . but the urea in the urine remains fairly constant. It is interesting to see people come here highly nervous, with great tension and with many wrinkles . . . and in a few days see a great change in their entire personality.

Urea and Wrinkles

Urea and wrinkles? This put a new "wrinkle" on the nutrition message of Dr. Reams. I could see all those Hollywood stars going through face-lifting operations to make them young again . . . and then only to face further face-lifting a couple years later.

When, if they would try a Reams urine/saliva test, follow the recommendations, drink only distilled water and follow a proper diet . . . their face might be young again . . . wrinkle-free. And not only their face, but their personality and their body could again be youthful.

Had I at last found the Fountain of Youth? From my experience at the retreat of Dr. Reams . . . although I am 51 . . . I now feel like 21! If I keep this up . . . I may be a teenager again!

(Please Print)

Name: CONNER ROBERT W.
     (Last)   (First)   (M.I.)

Address: 171 Peekskill Ave. SPRINGFIELD, MASS. 01129

Age: 55   Ht: 5' 9"   Wt: 160

Right Eye: _____   Left Eye: _____

Date	Sugar	pH	Saline	Albumen	Urea
3-17-76	5.4	$\frac{7.50}{7.60}$	28.C	4m	$\frac{10}{12}$
3-28-76	5.6	$\frac{6.80}{7}$	14.C	4m	$\frac{2}{9}$
3-29-76	1.2 0.8			4m	$\frac{1}{8}$
3-30-76	1.2 0.6			9m	$\frac{2}{8}$
3-31-76	4.6 0.6			4m	$\frac{1}{7}$
4-1-76	1.4	$\frac{5.60}{x}$	4.4C	4m	$\frac{1}{10}$
4-2-76	2.0			4m	$\frac{12}{12}$
4-3-76	2.8			4m	$\frac{9}{9}$
4-4-76	2.2			4m	$\frac{5}{8}$
4-6-76	4.8	$\frac{5.70}{x}$	26.C	4m	$\frac{11}{11}$
4-7-76	did'nt get specimen.				
4-8-76	2.2	$\frac{6.60}{x}$	12.C	4m	$\frac{4}{9}$

Actual final chart for Robert W. Conner at end of stay at the retreat which included a 3-day fast.

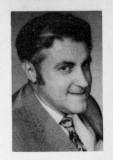

ROBERT W. CONNER
Health Analysis of Urine/Saliva Report

First Analysis/March 17, 1976

You are a prime candidate for a major heart attack.

You have a tendency towards low blood sugar,
 a fluctuating blood sugar.

Your food is digesting too slowly. You have headaches.

Your cholesterol is building up in the arteries and veins.

Your proteins are not digesting.

You have a little emphysema in both lungs.

You have some carcinoma in the prostate area and in the lower colon
and you have a minor hemorrhoidal condition.

Your reserve energy level is   **51.**

Analysis at end of fast and retreat schedule

You are no longer in the major heart attack zone.

On the second through sixth days your body went through withdrawal
and completed this on the eighth day.

Your digestion has improved considerably.

The cause of the cholesterol has dropped a little below normal. However, all of the cholesterol is not out yet. It is caused by the body retaining
too much salt.

Your report shows you are not drinking enough water.

You are allergic to white potatoes, tea, chocolate, spaghetti and macaroni.

You should eat meat only twice a week.

Your reserve energy level is now   **53.**

Name: KIRBAN, SAlem
　　　　(Last)　　　(First)　　(M.I.)

Address: 2117 Kent Rd. Huntingdon Valley, Pa. 19006

Age: 51　　　Ht: 5 10　　　Wt: 145

Right Eye: $(1-5)$ $(S-12)^+$　　　Left Eye: $(1-5)^+$, $(S-12)$

Date	Sugar	pH	Saline	Albumen	Urea
3-28-76	6.4	$\frac{6.20}{6.80}$	18.C	4 m	$\frac{10}{11}$
7-29-76	6.0 1.2			4m	$\frac{5}{8}$
3-30-76	5.0 2.4			4m	$\frac{1}{11}$
3-31-76	5.0 1.0			4m	$\frac{1}{10}$
4-1-76	3.0	$\frac{5.80}{x}$	12.C	4m	$\frac{2}{12}$
4-2-76	1.8			4m	$\frac{10}{12}$
4-3-76	4.2-2.4			4m	$\frac{12}{11}$
4-4-76	1.5			4m	$\frac{2}{10}$
4-6-76	4.0	$\frac{5.70}{x}$	20.C	4m	$\frac{10}{12}$
4-7-76	1.0			4m	$\frac{5}{8}$
4-8-76	1.0	$\frac{7.00}{x}$	6.8C	4m	$\frac{10}{4}$

Actual final chart for Salem Kirban at end of stay at the retreat which included a 3-day fast.

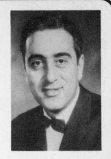

SALEM KIRBAN
Health Analysis of Urine/Saliva Report

First Analysis/March 28, 1976

You are in the zone for a minor heart attack.

You are a borderline diabetic.

The pancreas is not making enough insulin.
There is a deficiency in calciums that causes a little bit more inward tension.

The proteins are not digesting normally.

The cholesterol is building up in your system.

There is a little emphysema in both lungs and some carcinoma in the prostate area.

There is some carcinoma in the left kidney and a very little in the right kidney. There is also some in the left lobe of the colon.

Your reserve energy rating is   **48.**

Analysis at end of fast and retreat schedule

On the second day of your fast, your figures indicate you started into a body chemistry change which continued through the third and fourth day. On the fifth day you started coming out of the body chemistry change. On the last two days you have come completely out of this body chemistry change.

During this time the liver has needed a lot more calciums than we have given you because we want to know how much your body chemistry will do for itself.

Also these figures show that the pancreas is now manufacturing much more insulin than it was and it is almost functioning perfectly.

Your cholesterol has dropped about 30%. And that is a very good drop for this short length of time. You are out of the heart attack zone.

Your reserve energy level has now increased to   **54.**

(Author's note: After the fast I personally noticed that my allergy which plagued me for 8 months out of the year . . . suddenly disappeared. My energy seemed boundless. Prior to going to the retreat, I would arise about 8:30 every morning and rather tired. Now I arise at 6-7 each morning and full of energy. I can work straight through the day without tiring. The bottom of my feet, which were dry and scaly, are now smooth and tender. My sporadic indigestion and gas has completely disappeared!)

33

TRUTH IS STRANGER THAN FICTION

Will
Truth
Be Accepted?

How does one end a book like this? I wish that as you read this book you could have experienced the same experiences that I had at this mountain retreat.

One wise man once said:

Truth always lags behind, limping along on the arm of time.

Sir Isaac Newton was thrown in jail as an old man for insisting on the theory of the law of gravity.

The man who originally invented the telephone (and it was not Alexander Graham Bell) was thrown in jail for 20 years for his "heresy" that man could talk over wire.

Thomas Alva Edison at first suffered persecution for creating the electric light bulb.

Oliver Wendell Holmes wrote:

Sin has many tools, but a lie is the handle that fits them all.

I came here, up the winding dirt road of the Blue Ridge mountains, as a skeptic . . . an investigative reporter.

What I discovered was both heartwarming and sad. I met a man with a humble sense of dedication in applying principles of health which he felt were often found in the Bible . . . and applying them apparently successfully. In my opinion, with what appeared to be far, far, far greater success than the medical profession. I discovered that fully one-third of the Interfaith Church's budget is for the taking care of those who come without funds . . . worn by the years, sick in health, and in many cases, dying.

I was sad because I have seen the harassment of an arrest of Dr. Carey Reams at 2 AM. I was sad because I was again made aware of the know-it-all pride of men and organizations, who under the cloak of respectability, would exercise any possible avenue to prevent his continuing his life ministry of attempting to save and prolong lives.

I Have Seen the Dying in Hospitals

I have been in many hospitals. I have seen children dying. I have seen adults dying. I have seen them surrounded by a hardware array of pipes and tubes, suffering in agony from what may have been needless surgery, or dulled by deadly drugs.

Is there a better answer?

After writing this book the medical profession, (in my opinion), cannot continue to approach patients and offer them drugs or radiation or chemotherapy and not first at least investigate the alternative as suggested by Dr. Reams.

In my opinion, the medical profession can no

longer watch a child or a woman undergo radical surgery or die of leukemia or some other disease . . . and do nothing but administer drugs or recommend more surgery . . . unless they at least seriously study the route of the Reams method of a fast and individualized diet, and seek to find the answers as to why he has so often had success when the "doctors" have given up!

The physician may scoff at this book. The surgeon may call it a fraud . . . perpetuated to make money. I would challenge him to honestly and sincerely look into his own heart and bank account . . . to see what profession is making the most money.

It certainly will not be Dr. Carey Reams.

A Challenge to Disprove

I again recalled Dr. Reams telling me:

I welcome any study of my method and challenge them to disprove anything that I am doing.

Whenever one takes enough time and interest to make the tests, we have never been wrong!

In the television series, *The Upstairs Downstairs Maid*, the question is asked about World War 1:

What will history say?

The reply:

History, sir, will tell lies as usual.

What will history say of Dr. Carey Reams and his message of health and nutrition much of which he gleaned from the Biblical rules on food? I know not. I can only hope it will not be lies, but that the sunlight of truth may sear through the polluted doubts of the intelligensia and bathe the sick into a warmth of full recovery.

The Bible tells us that in the last days perilous times shall come and men shall be:

Ever learning, and never able to come to the knowledge of the truth. (2 Timothy 3:7)

**I Came
A Skeptic**

I came to the Blue Ridge mountains as a skeptic. I came to interview Dr. Carey Reams as an investigative reporter determined to report the facts as I saw them.

I have reported them as I saw and personally experienced them. You may draw your own conclusions.

After my eighth day at the Blue Ridge retreat of Interfaith Christian Church, I drove to Atlanta, Georgia to meet my wife who was coming to the retreat also.

We have been married 30 years.

She got off the plane, looked at me, then looked at me again and said:

You know, dear, I see a difference in you. You look just like when I first married you!

It was then I knew for sure, the message Dr. Reams gives is real.

**I Was
Alive
Again**

For the first time in my married life in years I was again alive, alert, peppy, and felt young once more. I had the energy of a teenager. The full vibrancy of youth had bloomed again! Life took on new meaning, new purpose. Actually, for the first time in my life I really understood life and knew what a healthy life was all about.

Those who have not experienced and followed the health message as proclaimed by Dr. Carey Reams may label Dr. Reams a quack and a charlatan and follow it up with medical mumbo jumbo.

But that is their <u>OPINION</u>!

But I know better! For I personally have been here at the retreat of Dr. Reams. I have gone through the 3-day fast and individualized diet recommendations. And I know that at least in my case what he said was true!

And that is <u>FACT</u>!

Dr. Carey Reams claims:

There is no such thing as an incurable disease!

And he believes that he can back this up by thousands of case histories of people who have taken a simple, inexpensive urine/saliva test and followed an individualized diet!

Let the Record SPEAK For Itself!

When and if ANYONE in the medical profession can make the same claim as Dr. Reams and have a similar track record of success as Dr. Carey Reams, I will be the first one to beat a path to his door and write a book on his successes.

Until that time, when the physicians come across a patient in which they have given up all hope . . . and want to offer a real service to that terminally ill dying soul . . . perhaps that doctor should have the courage and humility to suggest an alternative method recommended by Dr. Carey Reams.

And when the physician finds his own body

suddenly felled by a major illness, may he consider not just turning to the diffusion of drugs but rather also to God's door of diet.

You may disbelieve this book all you want. But you cannot disprove certain of the facts. **The simple things in life are often the hardest to believe.**

Somehow we feel more secure when illness strikes when we see a man in a white coat, with a stethescope, electrocardiagram machines, bustling nurses in white uniforms, the antiseptic smell of hospital rooms, the hushed quietness, that magic white prescription . . . somehow we are led to believe they will put us on the road to restored health.

The CHOICE IS YOURS

And then we go back again . . . back to waiting in doctor's waiting rooms, back to diagnostic tests . . . back to exploratory surgery, back to chemotherapy, back to inhalation therapy . . . back to radiotherapy . . . back to drugs until that very last drug and discover we are at the end of the line.

Or, in many cases we can try a urine/saliva test . . . if necessary go through a proper fasting procedure and then follow an individualized diet recommendation . . . and perhaps live!

The choice is yours.

Disbelieve all or part if you must!

But you owe it to yourself to honestly ask yourself the question:

Is my disbelief my opinion . . . or is it fact?

I can only direct you to what may be the

answer. But I cannot make you accept it. It's your life!

Yes, the choice is yours.

I have honestly reported an 8-day adventure into a strange land investigating another route for your **HEALTH GUIDE FOR SURVIVAL.**

And I am deeply indebted to Dr. Carey Reams.

For Dr. Reams showed me **HOW TO LIVE!**

Sequel to Fifth Edition

It has been 13 months since my stay at the Reams' Retreat in Blue Ridge, Georgia. How do I feel? I have never felt better in my life. At 52 years of age, I have greater vitality and energy than I did at 17! I have remained a constant 140 pounds; having lost 7 pounds during my 3-day lemon water fast. I arise earlier in the morning . . . wide awake without that usual tired feeling. I no longer experience fatigue during the day. My allergy has completely disappeared.

Robert Conner, who was 160 pounds, is now a trim 140 pounds and feels better for it. Prior to the retreat he averaged 2-3 migraine headaches *a week!* But in the last year he has only had one or two throughout the entire year . . . usually occurring when he strays off his nutritional program.

In the last year the Reams organization has been experiencing growing pains. Present plans are for starting an experimental farm in Murrieta California, where they have purchased a resort facility complete with mineral baths. Plans are to make this the Reams' headquarters. Laboratory technicians will also be trained in California. Many physicians are now looking into the Reams' Urine/Saliva technique and some have already enrolled in the Laboratory Technician classes taught by Dr. Carey Reams and Dr. John L. Black.